Family-Focused Treatment for Child and Adolescent Mental Health

This book is designed as a treatment manual for using family-based treatments with children struggling with mental illness, supporting both family therapists and the families they are helping.

Based on over 40 years of research, it has been shown that involving the entire family in treatment is effective. However, family therapy is still not used as a first line of treatment. Paul Sunseri explains and explores why family-based approaches should be used with struggling young people and how this can be applied in practice. Chapters discuss the causes, contributors, and social determinants for the rise in childhood mental illness and provide empirical evidence and treatments for working with children and adolescents suffering from self-harm, suicidal ideation, anxiety, anger, and depression. Filled with case studies throughout, the book also touches on mitigating the effects of screen time in our increasingly technological lives and interventions to help reluctant children participate in therapy. This book will be invaluable reading for graduate-level students, clinicians in training, and fully licensed clinicians, such as psychologists, psychiatrists, marriage and family therapists, and clinical social workers.

The book is also a practical resource for parents and other caregivers; it pulls back the curtain on therapy and teaches parents exactly what to do to best love and support their child at a time when they need it the most.

Paul Sunseri, PsyD, is a clinical psychologist who treats children and adolescents with serious mental health conditions. He has conducted research demonstrating the important role that families play in treating childhood mental illness. Dr. Sunseri is the developer of Intensive Family-Focused Therapy (IFFT), a family-based form of mental health care, in the United States.

Family-Focused Treatment for Child and Adolescent Mental Health

A New Paradigm

Paul Sunseri

Routledge
Taylor & Francis Group

NEW YORK AND LONDON

Designed cover image: © Getty Images

First published 2024
by Routledge
605 Third Avenue, New York, NY 10158

and by Routledge
4 Park Square, Milton Park, Abingdon, Oxon, OX14 4RN

Routledge is an imprint of the Taylor & Francis Group, an informa business

© 2024 Paul Sunseri

The right of Paul Sunseri to be identified as author of this work has been asserted in accordance with sections 77 and 78 of the Copyright, Designs and Patents Act 1988.

ISBN: 978-1-032-50199-4 (hbk)
ISBN: 978-1-032-50203-8 (pbk)
ISBN: 978-1-003-39736-6 (ebk)

DOI: 10.4324/9781003397366

Typeset in Sabon
by MPS Limited, Dehradun

"I did not realize how broken our healthcare system is until my daughter started to experience a serious mental health decline in her early teens. We were left to struggle through one of the biggest nightmares of our lives with very little help or guidance. This book is a must read for healthcare providers and for parents who feel lost with no light at the end of the tunnel."

G. Anderson, *Parent, USA*

"Working as a family to improve our daughter's mental health was absolutely critical. As parents, learning how to set boundaries, normalize our expectations, and communicate more effectively with her has had a far greater positive impact on her mental health than any individual child therapy in the past did. The treatment recommendations in this book have returned our daughter and family back into a healthy functioning dynamic."

J.C., *Parent, USA*

I am forever grateful to all of the families with whom I have had the honor and privilege of working. Everything I know I have learned from you.

And while I have truly loved many of these families, the one that is closest to my heart is, of course, my own. This book is dedicated to my amazing wife Vicki, and to our four daughters Katherine, Elisabeth, Taylor, and Olivia, who have grown up to become loving, strong, kind, compassionate, and fierce young women.

Contents

Introduction

Mental health challenges among young people are now a matter of national urgency.

The U.S. Surgeon General, Vivek Murthy, MD, states that we are in the midst of a mental health crisis for teens (Office of the U.S. Surgeon General, 2021). An increased trend toward higher rates of depression, anxiety, and suicide has been evident for the past decade, well before the onset of the COVID-19 pandemic. According to a CDC study, the suicide rate among adolescents and young adults was stable from 2000 to 2007, but increased 60% by 2018 (Curtin, 2020). With the onset of the pandemic, the situation is now far worse. Between March 2020 to October 2020, mental health-related emergency department visits increased by 24% for children ages five to 11 and by 31% for those ages 12 to 17 compared with 2019 emergency department visits (Leeb et al., 2020).

Now, more than ever, it is imperative that we identify and make available psychological treatments that work.

I am a clinical psychologist who specializes in the treatment of children and families. I wrote this book because I feel it is imperative that the mental health community change the way it is responding to the current crisis among young people. It is not through a lack of trying, of course. Dedicated, capable therapists, social workers, and psychiatrists all over the world are doing what they can. However, the gradual deterioration in well-being among children and adolescents continues to accelerate despite everyone's collective best efforts.

The problem is not with the therapy itself. Rather, most of the therapy is being aimed in the wrong direction in a manner entirely inconsistent with decades of research on how to best treat severe mental health challenges in children and adolescents.

There exists an implicit bias within the mental health system, in that most treatment is focused directly on the child or adolescent themselves. Most commonly, when a child begins to struggle in some way, parents are advised to send them to an individual therapist. The child or teen sits alone

DOI: 10.4324/9781003397366-1

in a room with a therapist, who theoretically says or does something that will help them feel better and hopefully behave differently. While in many cases, if the child's condition is mild or relatively uncomplicated, this is often sufficient. However, in more serious and challenging cases, for example, the young patients my colleagues and I see every day in our clinic, individual therapy alone has not helped them in the slightest. And, to make matters worse, when a child doesn't respond to individual therapy, we double down on an already bad idea by offering more individually-focused treatments. This includes sending them to an individualized outpatient program (IOP), a partial hospitalization program (PHP, which is really just the same thing as IOP but more hours per week), a psychiatric hospital, or a residential treatment program. While these types of programs can be valuable for some patients, they all make the same fundamental error—the belief that there is something going on inside the child that needs fixing.

I did a TEDx talk on this very subject, and I used an analogy that I will repeat here. Taking your child to see an individual therapist is like dropping them off for an oil change: "Please fix whatever's wrong with them and I'll be back in an hour."

It would be great if childhood mental health problems worked like that, but they simply do not. In my 40 years of clinical experience working with close to a thousand children and families, I've learned that the mental health community focuses far too much on what is happening on the inside of kids, i.e., their thoughts and feelings, and not nearly enough on what's happening to them on the outside. Thoughts and feelings are obviously important and should be attended to, but, in most cases, children and teens who begin to develop a mental health condition do so in response to the external influences or situational variables that are negatively affecting their emotional well-being. Through careful clinical assessment of what these influences and situational variables in the child's life are, each one in turn can be mitigated or buffered against. When this occurs, the child's mental health symptoms are vastly improved and their emotional well-being is greatly enhanced.

I believe that the reason individual therapy alone can often be ineffective is that even the best therapists lack the ability to disrupt or alter many of the situational variables that are having a negative impact on the child or teen. For example, I will be talking quite a bit throughout this book about the research demonstrating how excessive time on smartphones and other devices is a chief contributor to the decade-long decline in our children's mental health. Sure, an individual therapist can talk to a young patient about why it's good to take breaks from their phone, or why staying up too late on their phone causes sleep deprivation and how that affects their mood. However, even the most persuasive therapist lacks the power and influence to get kids to put their phones down. Or, if there are frequent conflicts or upsets within a family, which we know greatly impact a child's mental health, how can an individual therapist working in isolation do anything about that?

I can speak with some authority on individual therapy for children and teens because, honestly, I did just that for several years during the middle years of my practice. I wasn't really alone in this, as most therapists as a general rule don't do a lot of family therapy. Here is the honest truth of it—most therapists don't do family therapy because doing individual therapy is a lot easier. It is not particularly difficult, and often quite fun, to pass an hour with a 10-year-old. But an hour of therapy with kids and their parents together? That's a different story altogether. The therapist is juggling three or more different personalities who, in many cases, are hurt and angry, often reenacting the very conflicts in front of the therapist that take place at home. During a family therapy session, all hell can break loose unless the therapist works really hard to keep that from happening. Consequently, I didn't do a lot of family therapy either, but I quickly became very disillusioned with individual therapy, as I was clearly not being particularly helpful.

If treatments directed just at the child are often not effective, then what is? As it turns out, family therapy and family-based treatments have almost 40 years of research documenting their clinical efficacy, yet, surprisingly, they are not used as a first-line treatment for children and adolescents with serious mental health conditions. Family therapy tends to be an afterthought if it is thought of at all. The logic behind why family therapy might be more effective is not terribly surprising or complicated. If situational influences (things happening in a kid's external life) are negatively affecting their mental health, who is best positioned to mitigate or buffer against these influences than the child's parents? [*Note: I will be using the word parent or parents throughout this book only as a type of shorthand. I mean the words more broadly to include any primary caregiver in the child's life, such as grandparents, other extended family, foster parents, and so on.*] Unlike therapists, parents do have the power to reduce screen time, better insulate a child or teen from negative peer influences, reduce the amount of time a child or teen spends in their bedroom, and make use of skills to reduce conflict in the home by improving communication and peacefully solving problems as they arise.

In my practice, I tell parents that most of the positive changes in their child's functioning, i.e., improvements in their thoughts, feelings, and behavior, will be brought about by them and not by our clinical team. I see therapists as catalysts for change—we don't do most of the changing of the child directly ourselves, rather, we teach and empower parents to make changes at home that result in an improvement in their child's well-being. I have learned that when parents change the situation that changes the kid, it's really straightforward. In light of this, I want to focus my clinical attention on the people in the system who have the most power to bring about that change.

Furthermore, I feel strongly that good therapists work hard to make themselves obsolete in a family's life as quickly as possible. We should go in, do our work, and exit a family's life at the appropriate time, knowing that the changes we have brought about are sustainable over the family's lifetime. I tell parents that my ultimate goal is to help them have the closest, most loving relationship possible with their child, not just at this time in their lives, but forever.

Throughout this book, I will attempt to provide the reader with strong evidence that supports why a shift away from treatments directed primarily or exclusively at the child and toward more family-based interventions is the key to effectively addressing (and reversing) the current mental health crisis.

My background and the skill set I have acquired are somewhat unique. In addition to now being a family therapist, I am also a researcher who has studied the relationship between how well families get along and interact with each other and the severity of a child's mental health condition, which I will discuss in more detail later in the book. I am the developer of a model of family therapy called Intensive Family-Focused Therapy (IFFT), one of several family-based treatment models for children and adolescents. In this book, I will describe this model as well as other excellent family-based treatments.

I was fortunate enough to spend the early part of my career working in inpatient (residential) settings. Generally, children and teens are sent to residential treatment programs because their mental health conditions and associated behaviors are so severe that they cannot live successfully at home. At the time that I started (in the early 1980s), these programs were a bit like working in the Wild West of mental health. Little was known about how to best help a child who engaged in repeated self-harm, or children and teens who were highly oppositional and explosive. My job as a direct care staff member was to work with groups of children or teens to improve their behavior. I had no clue how to do this, and neither did any of the people with whom I worked. We all came into work and essentially fumbled around all day.

In truth, I learned by trial and error—mostly error. If a child did or said something that I wanted to change for the better (for example, cursing at me, hitting me, or hurting themselves), I would do or say something in response that I thought had a reasonable chance of making it less likely they would engage in that same behavior again. And trust me—these kids were *really hard*. A delight, but hard. Kids would break a light bulb and swallow the glass, jump off the roof, or think nothing of throwing a chair at me.

Their behavior problems were extensive and longstanding, so most of what I did simply didn't work at all. If I tried a response or intervention and it didn't work, I'd do my best not to use that intervention again, although I'm sure I made the same blunder repeatedly before I finally figured out what worked better.

However, here's what happened. These kids gradually shaped my own behavior. The outcome of a poorly conceived or executed response or intervention on my part was immediate and obvious—they'd usually just do more of what I didn't want them to do. However, if I did or said something that actually seemed to help and moved the needle in a positive direction, I would take note of that and try it again. I slowly learned what did and didn't work, and I gathered countless pieces of useful information about how to best help a child in distress. Many of these same interventions are what I teach parents and families to this day. In fact, I'm not sure I could do my job as a family therapist without all of those years of trial-by-fire learning.

Here's what I also learned during that time period in my life. *I love working with kids.* And hanging out with kids, talking with kids. They are the funniest and can be the most playful creatures on Earth, and they are just a joy to be around. I use a lot of playful humor with kids. Every kid has their own unique sense of humor, and once you find it and can make them laugh, it becomes an easy way to connect with them. I especially love really challenging, strong-willed kids. I've learned that kids can be in so much pain, hurting deeply, often behaving in ways that make no sense to adults, but in the end, they are just kids doing the best they can. They are often so lost, but they are relying on the only people who can pull them out of these dark periods in their lives—the people in their families who love them the most.

So, I've spent an awful lot of time with kids and their families, learning everything I can about them, and I have conducted research of my own to learn even more. I'm also a bit of a research junkie—I've done my best throughout this book to back up every idea that isn't my own with the relevant research findings to support my arguments.

This book serves two aims.

First, it is intended to be a treatment guide for clinicians (psychiatrists, psychologists, social workers, and other licensed psychotherapists) that provides numerous clinical techniques and interventions for those working to improve the mental health of children and teens.

Second, this book is written for parents as well, with the intention of being a guide or resource to them. If you are a parent who is not a clinician, and you are reading this book, you likely have a child or teen with a serious mental health condition. If you are at the beginning of that journey, I am certain that you are terrified, exhausted, under more stress than you ever imagined possible, and probably at a total loss as to how to help your child. I wrote this book so that you can better understand what treatments are available in order to access the best care possible for your child or teen. I have tried to write this book with a minimum of professional jargon, but if you end up having to do some Googling, then please accept my apologies in advance.

In addition, I am a great advocate of transparency in the field of psychotherapy. I feel my profession often does a poor job with this in ways that are not helpful for children and their families (more on this later). My hope is to pull back the curtain on what actually takes place in the therapist's office and why, and offer practical strategies you can use at home every day. I also believe that a book on family therapy should be written with parents in mind, not just therapists. It is in keeping with the spirit of family therapy: *We're all in this thing together.* Finally, in the very last chapter of this book, I will give you a number of practical, research-driven strategies that you can implement at home to improve your child's mental health.

The final chapter of the book also offers strategies for therapists and insurance companies that I believe stand at least some chance of reversing the upward trend of childhood mental illness.

Well, that's plenty of background stuff, I think. Let's get started and see what we can do to make the lives of children and their families a whole lot better.

References

Curtin, S. C. (2020). *State suicide rates among adolescents and young adults aged 10–24: United States, 2000–2018* (National Vital Statistics Reports, Volume 69, Number 11). U.S. Department of Health and Human Services, Centers for Disease Control and Prevention, National Center for Health Statistics, National Vital Statistics System. https://www.cdc.gov/nchs/data/nvsr/nvsr69/NVSR-69-11-508.pdf

Leeb, R. T., Bitsko, R. H., Radhakrishnan, L., Martinez, P., Njai, R., & Holland, K. M. (2020). Mental health-related emergency department visits among children aged <18 years during the COVID-19 pandemic — United States, January 1–October 17, 2020 (Morbidity and Mortality Weekly Report, Volume 69, Number 45). U.S. Department of Health and Human Services, Centers for Disease Control and Prevention. 10.15585/mmwr.mm6945a3

Office of the U.S. Surgeon General. (2021). *Protecting youth mental health: The U.S. surgeon general's advisory.* U.S. Department of Health and Human Services. https://www.hhs.gov/sites/default/files/surgeon-general-youth-mental-health-advisory.pdf

Part I

What In the World Is Going On and Where Does Change Begin?

1 Causes and Known Contributors to the Rise in Childhood Mental Illness

In this first chapter, I will provide a comprehensive overview of the likely contributing factors to the rise in mental health challenges among children and adolescents. Some of these will probably be familiar to you, but others will likely be a bit surprising. There has been considerable speculation as to why so many young people are suffering from depression, anxiety, and self-harm. This trend toward an increased prevalence of mental health problems in young people started to emerge in the year 2012, for reasons that we will discuss shortly.

Pediatricians, therapists, and psychiatrists are currently overwhelmed in their practices by what appears to be a massive wave of children and adolescents who are depressed, anxious, and suicidal. Parents are becoming increasingly worried that whatever is happening might lay claim to their own child, and, if it already has, they are at a loss as to what to do about it. We will start by looking at some obvious possible culprits: the effects of social media, bullying, and school shootings, and the role of COVID-induced social isolation. We will also consider two lesser-known influences that I believe play starring roles in all of this, but which are generally unknown or overlooked by parents and clinicians.

The Rise of Child and Adolescent Mental Health Challenges

The increasing prevalence of mental health challenges among children is well documented. One study found that major depressive episodes in adolescents ages 12 to 17 increased by 52% from 2005 to 2017 (Twenge et al., 2019). Another study found that emergency room visits among children and teens for suicidal thoughts and suicide attempts nearly doubled between 2008 and 2015, with adolescents between 12 and 17 displaying higher-than-average annual increases (Plemmons et al., 2018). Researcher Said Shahtahmasebi at the Center for Health and Social Practices states that despite heightened awareness of depression and mental illness and a

DOI: 10.4324/9781003397366-3

doubling of prescriptions for antidepressants, suicide rates have only continued to increase (Shahtahmasebi, 2013).

Younger girls and LGBTQ+ youth may be especially vulnerable to mental health struggles. Research indicates that the worldwide suicide rate for girls aged 10 to 14 has increased over the past two decades (Kõlves & De Leo, 2014). The Trevor Project's 2022 National Survey on LGBTQ Youth Mental Health found that in the previous year, 14% of LGBTQ youth ages 13 to 24 attempted suicide, and 45% of LGBTQ youth seriously considered attempting suicide (The Trevor Project, 2022). The survey also noted that 73% of LGBTQ youth reported experiencing anxiety symptoms and 58% reported experiencing depression symptoms. Living in a community that accepts LGBTQ people is a protective factor against suicide attempts, but fewer than 1 in 3 transgender and nonbinary youth reported that their home was gender-affirming.

U.S. Surgeon General, Dr. Vivek Murthy, has called for urgency in addressing the mental health crisis among the nation's youth, declaring that "mental health challenges in children, adolescents, and young adults are real and widespread" (Office of the U.S. Surgeon General, 2021). A study by the Centers for Disease Control and Prevention (Jones et al., 2022) reports that 42% of high school students "felt persistently sad or hopeless," with an alarming rate of 20% reporting having made a suicide plan in the past year. In the United States, the suicide rate among persons 10 to 24 years old was statistically stable from 2000 to 2007, then began to steadily rise (Curtin, 2020).

So what in the world is going on with our kids? Let's see what the evidence tells us.

Contributors to Mental Health Issues

The Effects of Digital Technology on Mental Health

I am going to be talking throughout this book about how spending excessive time on cell phones and other devices plays a significant role in the development and maintenance of mental health problems in children and teens. The importance of this cannot be overstated, and, later in the book I will discuss how reducing screen time is an essential component of providing effective treatment for reducing depression, anxiety, and suicide in our children.

According to the American Academy of Child and Adolescent Psychiatry (2020), adolescents currently spend up to nine hours a day on smartphones and other devices. The situation for younger children, ages eight to 12, is only slightly better but still alarming: four to six hours each day on a device. Our children's smartphones are, in essence, made to function as digital drugs—their number one purpose is to keep the user using, to generate as many advertising dollars as possible. Tech and social media companies market smartphones and advances in technology effectively to youth by portraying them as necessary. There is probably no more persuasive human being on the planet than an 11-year-old advocating for their first cell phone.

Researchers at the University of North Carolina at Chapel Hill gathered longitudinal data over the past several years focusing on the neurobiological effects of devices on brain development. They examined how technology use may be associated with changes in the adolescent brain and social development, including increased risk for behavioral health disorders such as depression and anxiety (Maza et al., 2023; Nick et al., 2022; Nesi et al., 2021).

Another study examined technology-based behaviors among adolescents, including comparing oneself with others and peer validation. As one might expect, social comparison and validation seeking were associated with increased depression. Some have suggested that the rise in mental health issues among girls is related to social media use because they are the heaviest users. Higher consumption of social media was found to be related to increased mental health issues compared with children and teens who engage in other activities that are "crowded out," such as sports, exercise, homework, and in-person social interaction (Twenge et al., 2018).

Fifty percent of teens reported that they "feel addicted" to mobile devices, while 59% of parents surveyed also believe that their children are addicted, according to a report by Common Sense Media in 2016 (Common Sense Media, 2016). Forty-five percent of teens said they use the internet "almost constantly," and another 44% said they go online several times a day, according to a Pew Research Report (Anderson & Jiang, 2018). Additionally, it reported that 50% of teenage girls are "near-constant" online users, compared with 39% of teenage boys. In the same report, it was also found that 43% of teenage cell phone users say they often or sometimes use their phones to avoid interacting with people. In addition, it was found that more than half of teens (56%) reported that the absence of their phone was associated with at least one of three emotions: loneliness, being upset, or feeling anxious. Girls were more likely than boys to feel anxious or lonely without their phones.

Another study examined adolescents' self-reported sleep duration and amount of time spent using electronic devices (Twenge et al., 2017). The study authors found that the reported sleep duration of U.S. adolescents decreased between 2009 and 2015, and that increased time spent on electronic devices is likely responsible for changes in sleep. Compared with 2009, adolescents in 2015 were 16% to 17% more likely to report sleeping fewer than seven hours a night on most nights. Children and teens who use electronic devices five or more hours a day were 50% more likely to experience short sleep duration (less than seven hours per night) compared with those spending one hour a day on devices (Twenge et al., 2017). Another study found that excessive cell phone use was a risk factor for insomnia (Tamura et al., 2017). In my own practice, it is common for parents to report their children are not falling asleep until very late at night, and that they are often quite difficult to wake up in the morning for school. On occasion, this is because the child reports feeling too anxious to fall asleep, but far more often they are up late on a device, often in secret. Lack of sleep is so important that it is one of the first things targeted for change with new families (more on how this is done later).

Cell phone use on social media sites may contribute to depression more than other activities on the internet, such as searching, playing games, or watching videos. One study examined the occurrence of problematic use of smartphones in a large sample of university students and the associated emotional and functional consequences of misuse (Grant et al., 2019). Twenty percent of the students sampled reported engaging in problematic cell phone use. Problematic use was associated with lower grade point averages and with alcohol use disorder symptoms. Problematic use was also significantly associated with impulsivity and elevated occurrence of PTSD, anxiety, and depression. Furthermore, an important study by Mingli Liu and her colleagues found a dose-related effect from the amount of time on a device: the risk of depression increases by 13% for each additional hour of social media use (Liu et al., 2022).

Here's what's important to know: social media per se is not the problem. Likely, for children and adolescents who have strong peer connections, interacting with those friends online and seeing pictures of oneself and them at some recent social event is undoubtedly a positive experience. However, for a child who has few friends, has difficulty keeping friends, or has just been painfully excluded from a group of friends, social media can be a source of great distress and sadness. *Everyone has a life but me.* These are the patients my colleagues and I typically see in our clinic—lonely, isolated, and excluded from the world. For a child or teen with a pre-existing vulnerability, for example, difficulty making and keeping friends, excessive time on devices appears to be a chief contributing factor to the development and maintenance of their mental health condition.

One final point on children and teenagers using smartphones and other devices. While the internet has obviously changed the world in many positive ways, giving children 24-hour access has, I believe, been a tragic mistake. Yes, it's great to be able to Google the major themes in *King Lear* when you're writing an essay for English class, but that is far from what they are doing. Smartphones are the gateway to the entire universe of human experience—the good, the bad, and the truly horrible. Decapitating someone held hostage by terrorists? Check. Mass graves of torture victims in Ukraine? Check. Pornography and every type of sexual behavior imaginable? Check. I do not think young people have the ability to make any real sense of the worst of human nature, but they are exposed to it well before they have the capacity to process and understand what they see. If, as a parent, I walked into my living room to find my 14-year-old watching a beheading on the TV screen, my reaction to this would be exactly as you'd expect. *Turn that off.* But this is what many of our kids are doing, alone in their bedrooms with no one to stop them or help them understand any of it.

You don't have to be a psychologist to know this must be having an effect on our children's mental health.

Bullying and Cyberbullying

Research shows that the experience of cybervictimization, or victimization that occurs through social media, is associated with heightened risk for suicide and self-injury. Bullying can increase the risk of suicidal ideation, not just for the victim but for the perpetrator as well (Holt et al., 2015; Quintana-Orts et al., 2019). A shocking 35% of adolescents report being bullied, and these experiences are associated with a two- to three-times increase in the rate of suicide ideation and suicide attempts (Modecki et al., 2014). One study examined the effects of being a victim of cyberbullying and its impact on suicidal thoughts and behaviors among youth. It was found that cyberbullying victimization increased suicidal thoughts by 14.5% and suicide attempts by 8.7% (Nikolaou, 2017). Perpetrators of cyberbullying, albeit to a lesser extent, are also at risk of suicidal behaviors and suicidal ideation when compared with non-perpetrators (John et al., 2018).

Prior to social media, bullying was primarily an in-person, awful experience. One needed to physically cross paths with the bully, thus limiting the frequency and duration of the mistreatment. Social media has changed all of that, allowing for the convenience of victimizing someone 24 hours a day. I find people are generally far braver behind a keyboard than in person, so social media can result in attacks being much more vicious and prolonged. It also makes it possible for other kids, also emboldened to some degree by the relative anonymity and physical distance, to pile onto a vulnerable child or adolescent, making the experience that much more sustained and brutal.

School Shootings and Active Shooter Drills

It comes as no surprise to anyone scrolling through their newsfeed that school shootings are on the rise. Shockingly, there is little in the way of research that has tried to understand the psychological effect of mass school shootings on children. The horrific events of Columbine took place in 1999, which means that every graduating senior, beginning from the year 2017, has gone to school in its shadow.

Active shooter drills and school lockdowns are now the reality of our children's educational experience. In previous generations, we practiced our own cohort's version of school-preparedness drills: "duck and covers" in the 1960s in case of an atomic bomb, and later, fire and earthquake drills. But these drills weren't particularly scary—we had no direct experience of these events actually occurring. No bombs were ever dropped, most students never experienced a serious earthquake, and fires in schools are rare. Since we never heard of any of these things occurring in our day-to-day lives, the drills themselves weren't particularly scary and we mostly just laughed our way through them.

But school shootings are very different. Every kid hears about them as soon as they occur, reads about the details of the shooting online, and talks about them at the dinner table with their parents who often don't know what to say. And the perpetrators of these horrific events are often *their own peers.* In between the shootings themselves, the active shooter drills (lights out, doors locked, saying nothing, and hoping for the best) and campus lockdowns regularly remind our children (not to mention their teachers) that they can be killed in their own classrooms and that the "precautions" offer no real measure of safety. How can any kid possibly make sense of this, and how can it not be having some sort of an impact on their mental health? Sadly, at least so far, no one knows.

COVID-19 and the Impact on Mental Health

The global pandemic has been a source of great distress all over the world. Social isolation, economic stressors, and the tragic loss of friends and loved ones have taken their toll on society in ways we are just now trying to understand. The impact of the pandemic on our children's well-being has been significant. Reduced access to mental health care and support services within schools and the community, along with fewer opportunities to engage in other protective activities (friends, sports, etc.) has negatively affected children's mental health (Marques de Miranda et al., 2020; Tsamakis et al., 2021, as cited in Chadi et al., 2022). The pandemic has been particularly damaging to youth with pre-existing vulnerabilities, such as children and teens experiencing high family adversity (Silliman Cohen & Bosk, 2020; Jones et al., 2020, as cited in Chadi et al., 2022).

During the pandemic, increased rates of financial and psychological distress were correlated with increased rates of suicide. In one study, researchers used real-time cellular phone location-tracking data and combined that with online search data from national databases

(Gimbrone et al., 2021). These data were then analyzed, and it was found that decreased mobility (spending more time at home) during the pandemic was associated with increased suicidality. Strong associations were also found between increased time spent at home and online suicide-related searches (e.g., "how to kill myself"). The data suggest that pandemic-related isolation, combined in many cases with acute economic distress, may be a risk factor for poor mental health and suicidal behavior. Similarly, in another study that also used geolocation-tracking information, for those diagnosed with major depressive disorder, more time spent at home was associated with greater severity of depressive symptoms (Laiou et al., 2022).

When I meet parents for the first time, it is very common for them to tell me that their child's mental health was often reasonably good prior to the onset of the pandemic. (Not all families, obviously). At that point, however, many parents observed a sharp decline in their child's functioning. Children and teens were spending significantly more time in their bedrooms and became depressed and less communicative. In addition, many kids took very poorly to online learning, and it was often a battle to get them to log into school and complete assignments. If you are a parent, you probably remember how hard this was. Parents report that their children were spending most waking hours on their phones, often until very late in the evening or early in the morning. Phones and social media became an even more vital conduit to the world for kids, both to stave off loneliness and as a way to pass the time, but what came with that was a corrosion of their mental well-being.

The pandemic was, therefore, a perfect storm. Rates of childhood mental health challenges had already been steadily increasing in the years prior. Shelter-in-place orders resulted in almost all time spent at home, and that factor alone could have triggered the onset of a child's depressed mood. Social isolation led to increased loneliness and few-to-no in-person social opportunities. Financial and other pandemic-related stressors also likely resulted in more conflict within families, which resulted in children and teens turning away from their parents while being pulled more toward negative online peer interactions. More time on a device means more time on social media, thus magnifying its negative effects. Mix up all those ingredients and you end up with a depressed teenager who spends far too much time on their phone and refuses to leave their bedroom.

Let's move our discussion to other possible causes responsible for the increase in depression, anxiety, and suicidal thoughts in children and teens. What follows are lesser-known and often overlooked influences, but in my judgment, they are vital to our understanding of what is happening and, ultimately, they are going to guide us in our clinical interventions.

Chief Takeaways from Chapter 1

For Parents

- While COVID-19 has made the situation worse, the trend toward increased depression, anxiety, and suicide in young people began well in advance.
- Younger teenage girls, LGBTQ+, and trans kids are especially vulnerable to developing mental health problems.
- Smartphones play an extremely important role in the epidemic of childhood mental illness, and their negative effects (and what to do about them) will be discussed in this book.
- For every additional hour on a device, the risk of depression increases by 13%.
- The world is a scarier place now than it was when you were growing up. Cyberbullying and school shootings are things your kids must cope with every day.

For Clinicians

- Become very knowledgeable about the negative impact of smart-phones and assess how much time your patients are spending online each day.
- Provide psychoeducation to your patients and their parents on the crowding-out effect (the tendency for devices to push away wellness-enhancing activities), along with the relationship between number of hours on a device and mood and overall well-being.
- Encourage and reinforce any attempts by kids to unplug and find more balance in their lives.
- If your patient has unrestricted access to their phone at night, it's really important that you assess whether they are getting enough sleep.
- If not, brainstorm as many ideas with them as you can to practice better device management at night.
- Share with parents what you've learned about your patient's device usage, and collaborate with them on how to reduce screen time.

References

American Academy of Child and Adolescent Psychiatry. (2020, February). *Screen time and children.* Retrieved May 4, 2023, from https://www.aacap.org/AACAP/Families_and_Youth/Facts_for_Families/FFF-Guide/Children-And-Watching-TV-054.aspx

Anderson, M., & Jiang, J. (2018, May 31). *Teens, social media and technology 2018.* Pew Research Center. https://www.pewresearch.org/internet/2018/05/31/teens-social-media-technology-2018/

Chadi, N., Castellanos-Ryan, N., & Geoffroy, M.-C. (2022). COVID-19 and the impacts on youth mental health: Emerging evidence from longitudinal studies. *Canadian Journal of Public Health, 113*(1), 44–52. 10.17269/s41997-021-00567-8

Centers for Disease Control and Prevention. (n.d.) *Mental health.* Retrieved May 9, 2023, from https://www.cdc.gov/healthyyouth/mental-health/index.htm

Common Sense Media. (2016, May 3). *New report finds teens feel addicted to their phones, causing tension at home* [Press release]. https://www.commonsensemedia.org/press-releases/new-report-finds-teens-feel-addicted-to-their-phones-causing-tension-at-home

Curtin, S. C. (2020). *State suicide rates among adolescents and young adults aged 10–24: United States, 2000–2018* (National Vital Statistics Reports, Volume 69, Number 11). U.S. Department of Health and Human Services, Centers for Disease Control and Prevention, National Center for Health Statistics, National Vital Statistics System. https://www.cdc.gov/nchs/data/nvsr/nvsr69/NVSR-69-11-508.pdf

Gimbrone, C., Rutherford, C., Kandula, S., Martínez-Alés, G., Shaman, J., Olfson, M., Gould, M. S., Pei, S., Galanti, M., & Keyes, K. M. (2021). Associations between COVID-19 mobility restrictions and economic, mental health, and suicide-related concerns in the U.S. using cellular phone GPS and Google search volume data. *PLoS One, 16*(12), Article e0260931. 10.1371/journal.pone.0260931

Grant, J. E., Lust, K., & Chamberlain, S. R. (2019). Problematic smartphone use associated with greater alcohol consumption, mental health issues, poorer academic performance, and impulsivity. *Journal of Behavioral Addictions, 8*(2), 335–342. 10.1556/2006.8.2019.32

Holt, M. K., Vivolo-Kantor, A. M., Polanin, J. R., Holland, K. M., DeGue, S., Matjasko, J. L., Wolfe, M., & Reid, G. (2015). Bullying and suicidal ideation and behaviors: A meta-analysis. *Pediatrics, 135*(2), e496–e509. 10.1542/peds.2014-1864

John, A., Glendenning, A. C., Marchant, A., Montgomery, P., Stewart, A., Wood, S., Lloyd, K., & Hawton, K. (2018). Self-harm, suicidal behaviours, and cyberbullying in children and young people: Systematic review. *Journal of Medical Internet Research, 20*(4), Article e129. 10.2196/jmir.9044

Jones, S. E., Ethier, K. A., Hertz, M., DeGue, S., Le , V. D., Thornton, J., Lim, C., Dittus, P. J., & Geda, S. (2022). Mental Health, Suicidality, and Connectedness Among High School Students During the COVID-19 Pandemic - Adolescent Behaviors and Experiences Survey, United States, January-June 2021. *MMWR Suppl, 71*(Suppl-3), 16–21. DOI: http://dx.doi.org/10.15585/mmwr.su7103a3 external icon

Kõlves, K., & De Leo, D. (2014). Suicide rates in children aged 10–14 years worldwide: Changes in the past two decades. *The British Journal of Psychiatry*, 205(4), 283–285. 10.1192/bjp.bp.114.144402

Laiou, P., Kaliukhovich, D. A., Folarin, A. A., Ranjan, Y., Rashid, Z., Conde, P., Stewart, C., Sun, S., Zhang, Y., Matcham, F., Ivan, A., Lavelle, G., Siddi, S., Lamers, F., Penninx, B. W. J. H., Haro, J. M., Annas, P., Cummins, N., Vairavan, S., ... the members of RADAR-CNS. (2022). The association between home stay and symptom severity in major depressive disorder: Preliminary findings from a multicenter observational study using geolocation data from smartphones. *Journal of Medical Internet Research mHealth and uHealth*, 10(1), Article e28095. 10.2196/28095

Liu, M., Kamper-DeMarco, K. E., Zhang, J., Xiao, J., Dong, D., & Xue, P. (2022). Time spent on social media and risk of depression in adolescents: A dose-response meta-analysis. *International Journal Environmental Research and Public Health*, 19(9), Article 5164. 10.3390/ijerph19095164

Marques de Miranda, D., da Silva Athanasio, B., Sena Oliveira, A. C., & Simoes-e-Silvac, A. C. (2020). How is COVID-19 pandemic impacting mental health of children and adolescents? *International Journal of Disaster Risk Reduction*, 51, Article 101845. 10.1016/j.ijdrr.2020.101845

Maza, M. T., Fox, K. A., Kwon, S.-J., Flannery, J. E., Lindquist, K. A., Prinstein, M. J., & Tezler, E. H. (2023). Association of habitual checking behaviors on social media with longitudinal functional brain development. *JAMA Pediatrics*, 177(2), 160–167. 10.1001/jamapediatrics.2022.4924

Modecki, K. L., Minchin, J., Harbaugh, A. G., Guerra, N. G., & Runions, K. C. (2014). Bullying prevalence across contexts: A meta-analysis measuring cyber and traditional bullying. *Journal of Adolescent Health*, 55(5), 602–611. 10.1016/j.jadohealth.2014.06.007

Nesi, J., Rothenberg, W. A., Bettis, A. H., Massing-Schaffer, M., Fox, K. A., Telzer, E. H., Lindquist, K. A., & Prinstein, M. J. (2021). Emotional responses to social media experiences among adolescents: Longitudinal associations with depressive symptoms. *Journal of Clinical Child and Adolescent Psychology*, 51(6), 907–922. 10.1080/15374416.2021.1955370

Nick, E. A., Kilic, Z., Nesi, J., Telzer, E. H., Lindquist, K. A., & Prinstein, M. J. (2022). Adolescent digital stress: Frequencies, correlates, and longitudinal association with depressive symptoms. *Journal of Adolescent Health*, 70(2), 336–339. 10.1016/j.jadohealth.2021.08.025

Nikolaou, D. (2017). Does cyberbullying impact youth suicidal behaviors? *Journal of Health Economics*, 56, 30–46. 10.1016/j.jhealeco.2017.09.009

Office of the U.S. Surgeon General. (2021). *Protecting youth mental health: The U.S. surgeon general's advisory*. U.S. Department of Health and Human Services. https://www.hhs.gov/sites/default/files/surgeon-general-youth-mental-health-advisory.pdf

Plemmons, G., Hall, M., Doupnik, S., Gay, J., Brown, C., Browning, W., Casey, R., Freundlich, K., Johnson, D. P., Lind, C., Rehm, K., Thomas, S., & Williams, D. (2018). Hospitalization for suicide ideation or attempt: 2008–2015. *Pediatrics*, 141(6), Article e20172426. 10.1542/peds.2017-2426

Quintana-Orts, C., Rey, L., Mérida-López, S., & Extremera, N. (2019). What bridges the gap between emotional intelligence and suicide risk in victims of bullying? A moderated mediation study. *Journal of Affective Disorders, 245,* 798–805. 10.1016/j.jad.2018.11.030

Shahtahmasebi, S. (2013). De-politicizing youth suicide prevention. *Frontiers in Pediatrics, 1,* Article 8. 10.3389/fped.2013.00008

Silliman Cohen, R. I., & Bosk, E. A. (2020). Vulnerable youth and the COVID-19 pandemic. *Pediatrics, 146*(1), Article e20201306. 10.1542/peds.2020-1306. Epub 2020 Apr 28. PMID: 32345686.

Tamura, H., Nishida, T., Tsuji, A., & Sakakibara, H. (2017). Association between excessive use of mobile phone and insomnia and depression among Japanese adolescents. *International Journal of Environmental Research and Public Health, 14*(7), Article 701. 10.3390/ijerph14070701

The Trevor Project. (2022). *2022 national survey on LGBTQ youth mental health.* https://www.thetrevorproject.org/survey-2022/assets/static/trevor01_2022survey_final.pdf

Twenge, J. M., Krizan, Z., & Hisler, G. (2017). Decreases in self-reported sleep duration among U.S. adolescents 2009-2015 and association with new media screen time. *Sleep Medicine, 39,* 47–53. 10.1016/j.sleep.2017.08.013

Twenge, J. M., Joiner, T. E., Rogers, M. L., & Martin, G. N. (2018). Increases in depressive symptoms, suicide-related outcomes, and suicide rates among U.S. adolescents after 2010 and links to increased new media screen time. *Clinical Psychological Science, 6*(1), 3–17. 10.1177/2167702617723376

Twenge, J. M., Cooper, A. B., Joiner, T. E., Duffy, M. E., & Binau, S. G. (2019). Age, period, and cohort trends in mood disorder indicators and suicide-related outcomes in a nationally representative dataset, 2005-2017. *Journal of Abnormal Psychology, 128*(3), 185–199. 10.1037/abn0000410

2 Lesser Known but Likely More Impactful Causes and Contributors

The Curious Case of Micronesia

In Micronesia, a country consisting of approximately 2,000 small islands in the western Pacific Ocean, suicide among adolescents and young adults was relatively unknown prior to the early 1960s. In his excellent book, *The Tipping Point*, Malcolm Gladwell discusses Micronesia's rapid increase in suicide and why it is worth our attention (Gladwell, 2006).

Suicide rates dramatically increased during the time period in which Micronesia became more modernized due to a program initiated by the United States in the early 1960s and continuing into the 1980s. By that time, rates of suicide among adolescent boys in Micronesia were seven times higher than the suicide rate in the United States. Suicide rates peaked in the early 1980s but remained elevated compared with the global averages well into the 2000s (Lowe, 2019).

Suicides in Micronesia had oddly similar characteristics. Dying by suicide occurred primarily among adolescent boys and young adult men, often triggered by some seemingly minor event such as an argument with a family member or romantic partner. For example, some boys took their lives because their father yelled at them, because they saw their love interest with someone else, or because their parents refused them some small request. One 19-year-old hanged himself because his parents didn't buy him a graduation gown, and a 17-year-old also hanged himself because his older brother chastised him for making too much noise. The suicides tended to follow a similar, almost scripted pattern: males only, in late teens or early 20s, a precipitating event related to upsets with a girlfriend or parent, suicide notes that expressed both unhappiness and what can be best characterized as "wounded pride," the act itself done in a remote spot, and death by hanging. The hanging itself followed a specific protocol: the noose was tied on a low branch or window with the child leaning forward. In three-quarters of cases, the child had never attempted suicide before, or even spoken about suicidal intent (Gladwell, 2006).

DOI: 10.4324/9781003397366-4

Suicide often occurred among those who knew each other, and upon hearing of one suicide, others seemed to have been given permission to do the same. The clustering of suicides was a distinctive feature in the region. On one island, the death of a prominent political figure triggered a number of suicides in the following months. Clusters of suicide victims tended to occur in a single village during a short time frame (Rubinstein, 1987, as cited in Twaddle et al., 2022, Chapter 1).

So what did social scientists make of all this? A "social disintegration hypothesis" was proposed, and it asserted that the increased suicide rates reflected a decline in family-based activities and community institutions. Another hypothesis proposed was that the young men struggled with conflicting values reflected by popular culture and in the media regarding the importance of material wealth in a way that conflicted with traditional family values (Lowe, 2019).

I suppose maybe, yes, it makes sense that when previously well-connected families are now less connected it might have an effect on a child's well-being (a family therapist is never going to argue otherwise), or if institutions have become eroded and a cultural perspective on material wealth has shifted. Common sense, however, tells you that these proposed causal explanations fall well short of accounting for all the startling similarities in the circumstances surrounding the deaths of these young men—age, gender, wounded pride, clusters of suicides in the same village, choosing a remote location, death by hanging, and so on. If it were just a matter of social disintegration, one would expect more variability in the manner in which someone would take their life, but that is not the case.

What is occurring among these young men is obvious: they are imitating each other. Suicidal behavior became contagious and spread through the young male population.

Suggestibility and Social Contagion

The Social Contagion Hypothesis

One of the hallmarks of our species, and of most non-human primates, is our highly social nature and the corresponding relational complexities that exist between ourselves and others. We share a common belief (or maybe the illusion) that as individuals our behavior is driven more or less by our own thoughts, emotions, needs, and desires, and that while the behavior of others in our social environment might affect us to some degree, we ourselves—as individuals—are largely in the driver's seat.

I am not sure this is necessarily the case, or at least not to the extent we would all like to believe. There exists a well-established body of research that has examined the phenomenon known as social contagion.

Origins the of Social (Behavioral) Contagion Hypothesis

The term, "behavioral contagion" was first coined by a French polymath (think "renaissance man") by the name of Gustave Le Bon in his 1895 book *The Crowd: A Study of the Popular Mind* (Le Bon, 1895/1896). Le Bon asserted that behaviors are contagious (imitated) in social populations. He argued that feelings and behaviors are contagious to such a degree that an individual readily sacrifices his personal interests for the collective interest. Robert Park later revised Le Bon's theory. Park asserted that during times of stress, people are more attuned to each other than they normally would be, so the thoughts and behaviors of each member of the group influence each other in a circular way. Park asserted that when in a crowd under high stress, people can sometimes lose their ability to think logically and rationally and begin to mindlessly imitate each other (Locher, 2002). If you've ever watched an agitated post-game crowd destroy entire city blocks, then you'll understand what Park had in mind.

Herbert Blumer (1939) defined social contagion as something that spreads rapidly, impulsively, and unconsciously. Blumer asserted that social contagion is likely to take place when collective excitement is intense and widespread, which, in turn, is then transmitted to bystanders. Blumer asserted that people observe reactions in others and develop similar reactions within themselves.

The social contagion hypothesis argues that behaviors and attitudes are like a virus that is transmissible within social groups. The acceptance and adoption of certain behaviors can and are passed from one person to another with surprising ease (Purington & Whitlock, 2010). Emotional contagion, an offshoot of social contagion, has been defined as "The tendency to automatically mimic and synchronize expressions, vocalizations, postures, and movements with ... another person's and, consequently, to converge emotionally" (what I refer to as "mirroring and matching," to be discussed later in the book) (Hatfield et al., 1993). Adolescents tend to be more affected by social contagion, largely due to being in the stage of identity formation. This makes them more vulnerable to social influences including peer pressure, social expectations, and aspirations (Papadima, 2019). Young people also tend to be more suggestible and, therefore, more vulnerable to the influence of social contagion (Gould, 2001).

Social Networks and Contagion

Numerous, and sometimes very surprising, behaviors have been identified that are susceptible to social contagion. One study examined poor sleep and drug use among adolescents and concluded that both could be spread through social networks (Mednick et al., 2010). Adolescents who were in a large social network with those who had poor sleep and used drugs were more likely to struggle with both problems themselves. Quite astonishingly, the effects of poor sleep and drug use extended up to four degrees of separation (to one's friends' friends' friends' friends) before the effects began to diminish.

Another study examined whether alcohol consumption could spread through large social networks. It was found that changes in the amount of consumption of alcohol in one's social network group predicted an individual's changes in alcohol consumption in the future. This effect held for up to three degrees of separation before diminishing (Rosenquist et al., 2010).

Researchers Nicholas Christakis and James Fowler have extensively studied how behaviors and emotions spread within social networks. For example, obesity is subject to social influence. Christakis and Fowler (2007) evaluated a densely interconnected social network of 12,067 people assessed repeatedly from 1971 to 2003. They found that a person's chances of becoming obese increased if someone in their social network became obese in that same time period. For example, if your friends are obese, your risk of being obese is 45% higher. The clusters also extended up to three degrees of separation. The effects were not the result of obese people choosing friends who were also obese. For an excellent overview of their work on understanding social and emotional contagion, I highly recommend watching Christakis's 2010 TED talk "The Hidden Influence of Social Networks."

Loneliness can also spread via social contagion. A study found that people who are lonely tend to be linked to others who are also lonely, an effect that is stronger for friends who live closer geographically than distant friends (Cacioppo et al., 2009). The nature of the friendship matters, as well, in that nearby mutual friends show stronger effects than nearby ordinary friends. Analyses also indicated that non-lonely individuals who are around lonely individuals tend to grow lonelier over time. The link to loneliness extended to up to three degrees of separation. These data also support the contagion effect rather than lonely individuals preferring friends who are also lonely.

Mass Psychogenic Illness: Fainting spells, Tics, and More

Mass psychogenic illness (formerly called mass hysteria) is an intriguing phenomenon with numerous examples occurring throughout history. It often begins with people of a particular group who start to believe that they might have been exposed to something dangerous, such as bacteria, a virus, or a poison. They believe the threat to be real because others say so, and begin to experience the same symptoms.

One of the earliest examples of mass hysteria occurred during the Middle Ages at a time when many were dying of the bubonic plague.

Groups of people within a town struck by the plague would dance, shriek, scream, and convulse in a manner unrelated to the illness itself. These symptoms would then pass from groups of people from one town to the next. It was theorized that the stress of the plague, as well as grief, made people vulnerable to social contagion (Hatfield et al., 2014).

Another notable and more recent example of mass hysteria occurred at Warren County High School in McMinnville, Tennessee in November 1988. After a teacher reported smelling a "gasoline-like smell" in her classroom, a total of 100 students and staff members went to the local ER with symptoms they believed were related to the supposed exposure. Symptoms occurred suddenly, and included headache, nausea, dizziness, and shortness of breath. However, toxicology reports indicated no exposure to harmful substances. Several governmental agencies conducted investigations of the environment and found nothing to explain the symptoms (Jones et al., 2000).

Another example of mass hysteria occurred in the country of Jordan in 1998. Eight hundred young people reported symptoms of headache and dizziness after being vaccinated for tetanus. After some students were vaccinated, the other students waiting in line observed symptoms of illness in those vaccinated and reported symptoms themselves. However, investigations revealed that the effects were not related to the vaccine itself, as no other reports of illness occurred in other vaccine locations (Kharabsheh et al., 2001).

A more recent example of mass psychogenic illness, the first one likely spread through social media, started in Tapachula, Mexico (Perlmutter, 2023). Twelve students in a middle school fainted at the same time. Two weeks later in another middle school 150 miles away, 68 students also fainted. Over the next two months, mass fainting was reported in six other middle schools in four Mexican states, separated by hundreds of miles, affecting a total of 227 children. It was initially thought that each school was unconnected to the others until it was learned that news of the fainting incidents was being spread by students on WhatsApp.

The rapid onset of tic-like symptoms among adolescents during the pandemic is another fascinating example of mass psychogenic illness. For example, Tourette syndrome is a neurological condition that begins in childhood, characterized by sudden, uncontrolled movements or sounds. Tics can include blinking or clearing one's throat over and over again or blurting out sounds or inappropriate words. Pediatricians began to notice a sudden increase in young patients presenting with tics, mostly adolescent girls. Onset was rapid, patients had no prior history of tics, and the tics themselves did not fit the typical profile of those with Tourette's. These patients were ultimately diagnosed with functional tic-like disorder

(FTLD) after having watched numerous TikTok videos of other girls displaying their own tic-like behaviors. One study theorized that the increase in the number of videos of those displaying tics, combined with the stress associated with COVID-induced social isolation, led to the increase in FTLD (Heyman et al., 2021). In her book, *The Sleeping Beauties: And Other Stories of Mystery Illness*, neurologist Suzanne O'Sullivan (2021) describes a number of interesting functional disorders that can be found throughout the world today. A functional disorder is one for which the patient's symptoms have no biological basis but serve a purpose of some kind, often on an unconscious level. Many of the symptoms and behaviors I see in my patients clearly serve a function, which I will talk more about later in the book.

Social Contagion and Depression

A review of studies regarding social contagion and depression has found that depressed people can induce negative moods in others through social interaction (Segrin & Dillard, 1992). Peer contagion processes are relevant for symptoms of depression. Studies have identified depression symptom contagion between mothers and children. It was found that children who had depressed mothers were more likely to be depressed themselves. Children who were experiencing high stress but did not have depressed mothers were less likely to be depressed (Hammen et al., 1991).

Another study was conducted to measure depression among college roommates and to determine if symptoms of depression can be socially transmitted. As predicted, roommates of depressed students became more depressed themselves over the course of the study (Joiner, 1994). The effect persisted when the existing levels of depression at the start of the study and negative life events experienced by roommates were considered In another study, it was found that persons without depression who interacted with depressed persons for 15 minutes became more depressed, anxious, and hostile themselves after the interaction (Strack & Coyne, 1983).

Depression can be socially transmitted within dating couples. One study found that someone dating a depressed person was much more likely to be depressed themselves, even when controlling for relationship satisfaction and pre-existing levels of depression (Katz et al., 1999). Depressive symptoms within established couples also appear to be socially contagious. A study investigated 11,136 couples over a 12-year period. Depressive symptoms were measured across time for each member of the couple. It was found that individuals' mental health became more similar to their partners over time. If one member of the couple experienced a change in their mental health, then the other member was increasingly likely to experience a similar change in their own mental health. It was found that depressive symptoms in one partner often led to depressive symptoms in the other partner over time (Walters, 2022).

In another study, female adolescents who have a best friend who is depressed are more likely to experience depression themselves (Stevens & Prinstein, 2005). Hogue and Steinberg (1995) also suggest that adolescents who were friends with someone with depression were associated with changes in the adolescents' own self-reported depressive symptoms over time.

Social Contagion and Anxiety

Anxiety can also be transmitted through social contagion. Catherine Serra Poirier and her colleagues hypothesized that anxiety can be transmitted between twin siblings. It was found that after controlling for genetic factors, stress, and the quality of the relationship, if one twin experiences anxiety symptoms the other twin is more likely to have anxiety symptoms as well. The closer the relationship between the siblings, the increased likelihood that if one twin reported symptoms of anxiety the other twin would also report symptoms of anxiety. It was theorized that social contagion of anxiety was to blame and that close relationships may make it more likely for social contagion to occur (Serra Poirier et al., 2017).

Another study found that symptoms of anxiety and depression were the result of social contagion among adolescent friends and that symptoms of anxiety were the result of social contagion among adolescent female friends, but not male. It was theorized that female friends may express more negative affect and talk about their problems with each other, which makes symptoms more likely to spread via social contagion, compared with male friends who may not express negative affect and discuss problems with each other (Schwartz-Mette & Rose, 2012).

Another study also investigated whether social anxiety could be transmitted to others via emotional contagion. Participants in the study watched a video presenter who seemed socially anxious or watched a video of a non-anxious presenter. After controlling for baseline anxiety levels, participants who watched a video of a socially anxious presenter reported significantly higher levels of anxiety during and immediately after watching the video compared with individuals who watched the video of the non-anxious presenter (Shaw et al., 2021).

Social Contagion and Self-Injury

There is growing evidence that suggests social media can influence suicide-related behavior by way of social contagion (Purington & Whitlock, 2010). One study explored the influence of Facebook on mental health, nonsuicidal self-injury, and suicidal behavior in college students. For some individuals, Facebook can lead to more self-injurious behavior, such as cutting. Another study investigated the effects of joining a group for nonsuicidal self-harm on Facebook. Members of one self-harm discussion group completed a web-based questionnaire. It was found that many participants in nonsuicidal self-injury groups on Facebook found the groups to be beneficial, and 73% said these groups led to a decrease in nonsuicidal self-injury. However, this same study found that 11% of respondents attributed these groups to an increase in their self-injurious behavior (Murray & Fox, 2006).

At least at this moment in time, in my experience, Instagram seems to be one of the most popular social media platforms among adolescents. Pictures and communication about nonsuicidal self-injury can be easily found on Instagram. Researchers found that people who self-injure often post pictures of their injuries, frequently resulting in empathic comments from others (Brown et al., 2018). The more serious the injury, the more empathic comments they received, which very likely reinforced (made stronger) the behavior. Similarly, Nock and Prinstein (2004) state that social reinforcement is an important factor in nonsuicidal self-injury. Posting pictures of injuries online might also provide positive social reinforcement through feedback received in the form of comments or likes for pictures of nonsuicidal self-injury.

A study investigating self-harm and social influence on Instagram also showed that nonsuicidal self-injury can be socially contagious (Jarvi et al., 2013). It found that pictures on Instagram of nonsuicidal self-injury might put adolescents at risk of initiating this behavior or it might be triggering for users already engaging in self-injury (Baker & Lewis, 2013). In another study, analyses were conducted on exposure to self-harm on Instagram and the emotional ramifications that occur. It found that exposure to self-harm on Instagram was associated with suicidal ideation, self-harm, and emotional disturbance (Arendt et al., 2019).

Influence of Media on Suicide Attempts

Exposure to media depictions of suicide can cause those who consume such media to imitate these suicides, which may lead to additional suicides (Romer et al., 2006; Stack, 2005). Interviews were conducted with adolescents who attempted suicide. It was found that high exposure to suicide-related events, such as having relatives who died by suicide and watching actors on TV depict suicide, can induce suicidal behaviors in vulnerable adolescents (Bazrafshan et al., 2016). Another study examined the association between reporting on suicides, especially deaths of celebrities by suicide, and subsequent suicides in the general population. The risk of suicide increased by 13% in the period after the media reported the death of a celebrity by suicide. When the suicide method used by the celebrity was reported, there was an associated 30% increase in suicides by the same method (Niederkrotenthaler et al., 2020). Research shows that individuals with a recent history of a suicide attempt or severe depression are more likely to attempt suicide after a media report of suicide (Gould et al., 2014). In another study, patients with depression were interviewed after a celebrity suicide was extensively covered by the media. It was found that 38.8% of patients reported that the media coverage of the suicide influenced their suicidal behaviors, with 5.5% of patients reporting that it influenced their suicide attempt. The risk was the highest for those who had attempted suicide one month prior to the media coverage (Cheng et al., 2007).

Suicide Clusters

Suicide clusters are of two main types, mass clusters and point clusters. Mass clusters are media-related phenomena where suicides occur during a short period following, and linked to, the broadcasting or publishing of actual or fictional suicides. Point clusters, also known as space-time clusters, are when an unusually high number of suicides occur in a small geographical area or institution over a brief period. Point-clustered suicides may occur when people are exposed to triggering stimuli—including a severe negative life event, such as the suicide of a peer—and, if vulnerable due to lack of social support, simultaneously develop suicidal symptoms (Joiner, 1999). This study involved studying the suicide rates at three primary schools after the suicides of five students occurred. It was hypothesized that, after the suicides, other students at the same school were at increased risk for suicide. The study found a much higher probability for those students to commit suicide compared with the general population of the same age. In this study, the time interval from the death of the student before a new suicide of a student took place was one to four months. The method of the suicides also seemed to be an imitation of the first students' suicides. All of the victims of the second wave of suicides knew about the suicide, had been friends of the student who committed the initial suicide, and knew about the method of suicide (Poijula et al., 2001).

Approximately 1–5% of teen suicides occur in a cluster after a youth dies by suicide (Gould & Lake, 2013, p. 70). A cluster, as defined by the Centers for Disease Control, is when multiple suicides occur close in time and geographical area at a rate greater than normally would be expected in a given community (National Center for Injury Prevention and Control, n.d.). Clustering was two to four times more common among adolescents and young adults than among other age groups (Gould et al., 1990). Exposure to a peer's suicide has been found to be associated with suicidal ideation or behavior in adolescents and can persist for up to two years among vulnerable adolescents. Factors that make adolescents vulnerable to suicidal ideation or behaviors include current or past psychiatric conditions, family history of suicide, past suicide attempts, substance abuse, stressful life events, access to lethal methods, incarceration, social impairments, environmental factors, and lack of protective factors (Gould et al., 2018).

Helicopter Parenting and the Loss of Independence

Twenge (2017) argues that the world is now safer for children and adolescents than at any other time in human history. Relative to previous generations, today's children and teens are kept safer by being more carefully supervised, not being allowed to play freely in their neighborhoods, not walking or biking to school on their own, and being taught to be cautious of strangers. The current generation of teenagers, Generation Z, and soon their successors, Generation Alpha, have grown up in a world in which they are watched far more closely by substantially more involved parents than any previous generation.

This societal shift toward a focus on safety and involvement coincides with a style of parenting commonly referred to as "helicopter parenting." The term "helicopter parent" was first coined in 1990 by Foster Cline and Jim Fay in their book, *Parenting with Love and Logic* (Cline & Fay, 1990, as cited in Schwartz, 2018). While coming from a place of deep love and affection, helicopter parents tend to be overly protective and involved in their children's lives. Deepika Srivastav and M. N. Lal Mathur describe helicopter parenting as overly protective, highly intensive, and highly involved with the children (Srivastav & Lal Mathur, 2021).

Helicopter parenting can be identified by three main qualities: information seeking, direct intervention, and autonomy limiting (Luebbe, 2018). Samuel Hunley of Emory University gives typical examples of helicopter parenting, such as knowing the child or teen's daily schedule, knowing their whereabouts at all times (by tracking their phone), and helping them make everyday decisions. Other behaviors might include directly intervening in disputes with teachers, roommates, friends, romantic partners, and so on (Hunley, 2017). These types of parenting strategies would have been unheard of in previous generations.

Effects of Helicopter Parenting on Adolescent Functioning

Research by Neil Montgomery (2010) at Keene State College suggests that overprotective parenting may have long-term effects on the child's personality by prolonging childhood and adolescence. He studied a group of 300 college freshmen and found that students with helicopter parents "tended to be less open to new ideas and actions, and were more vulnerable, anxious, dependent, and self-conscious." Without the opportunity to make mistakes during childhood, teens are ill-prepared to enter adulthood, as they've often had little or no practice at making independent decisions.

Hayley Love (2019) and her colleagues found that helicopter parenting "may hinder the development of self-control skills among emerging adult college students, which are associated with feelings of school burnout." Additionally, helicopter parenting has been associated with a multitude of difficulties: problems with emotional regulation, academic productivity, and social skills, as well as a lack of trust in and alienation from peers, and low self-efficacy (Srivastav & Lal Mathur, 2021). While helicopter parenting may give the illusion of protection in the short term, the reality is that these children can grow up to become adults who struggle with functioning in everyday areas of life, such as work, school, and relationships.

Similarly, Aaron Luebbe (Luebbe et al., 2018) and his colleagues found that helicopter parenting was "associated with poorer functioning in emotional functioning, decision making, and academic functioning." Nevertheless, the researchers also found that "information-seeking behaviors, when done in absences of other [helicopter parenting] behaviors, were associated with better decision making and academic functioning." That is, parents knowing about their child's life without becoming overly involved was linked to more positive outcomes.

In a commentary published in the *Journal of Pediatrics*, Peter Gray and his colleagues make a compelling argument that the rise in depression, anxiety, and self-harm in children and teens coincides with the decline in providing opportunities for engaging in independent activities (Gray et al., 2023). These opportunities include time spent playing without direct adult supervision, taking age-appropriate risks (such as climbing trees for example), making meaningful contributions to the family (helping out around the house), and taking on adult responsibilities such as getting a driver's license and a part-time job.

Statistical data supports a decline among Gen Z in these activities, which were common in previous generations. For example, fewer and fewer teens are getting their driver's licenses. In 1983, 46.2% of 16-year-olds had their driver's license but by 2018, that number dropped down to 25.6% (Federal Highway Administration, 2020). In fact, in 2018, only 60.9% of 18-year-olds had their driver's license. In my practice, I rarely see adolescents who have their driver's license, and when I ask why, I most often hear, "The thought of that makes me anxious." They are even less likely to have a part-time job. According to the Bureau of Labor Statistics, among teens aged 16–19 in the United States, the percentage who had part-time jobs fell from a high of 31% in 1998 to a low of 17.6% in 2020 (Duffin, 2023). Furthermore, in a survey of 1,001 U.S. adults, conducted by Braun Research, 82% reported having regular chores growing up, but only 28% said that they require their own children to do them (Wallace, 2015). This survey was conducted in 2015, so I suspect the number is even lower now. So, we have this ultra-protected generation growing in much safer environments, and being asked to do less and less, but we also have far more anxious and depressed kids.

Learning how to do hard things without relying on parents for support is a key factor in developing resilience. Pause for a moment and think about all of the skills that are learned in getting a job for the first time. Kids have to show up on time, work in sometimes less than pleasant environments, follow orders from a manager barely older than themselves, interact with abrasive co-workers or customers, and learn how to stay emotionally well-regulated while under stress.

Please note that I am not proposing that we move back in the direction of previous styles of parenting. The Silent Generation of parenting, that is the parents of the Baby Boomers, were far less involved in their kids' lives and much less attuned to their children's inner thoughts and feelings. I can say this with some confidence because that's the generation that parented me, and it is a common topic among my same-age Baby Boomer friends as to how distant and disconnected our parents were. If my parents or the parents of any of my friends threw a party, we were expected to make a brief appearance (maybe) and then not be seen again. When I was at a sleepover, I don't recall ever seeing a parent in the vicinity, which suited us just fine. (For an interesting and highly entertaining comparison to sleepovers today, see "Sleepovers are now a Battleground" [Florsheim, 2023].)

To say the least, this was not what anyone would likely characterize as ideal parenting. I recall making a conscious decision when I was young to be a different, much more involved and connected parent, as I suspect most Baby Boomers did. Evidence of this societal shift became apparent in the 1980s, with movies and television depicting this new breed of more involved parents—fathers especially. Some might still remember the "Baby on Board" placards, which I'm certain my own parents' generation found quite puzzling.

Being a more attentive and engaged parent is obviously a positive change, but as is often the case, too much of a good thing quality is no longer a good quality. It also appears that the current cohort of parents has fallen into some sort of parenting arms race to see who can be the most "protective" (or engage in virtue signaling by talking about not having enough hours in the day to shuttle their kids from one extracurricular activity to another). I will be curious to see how Gen Z and Gen Alpha parent their own children, but I would not be at all surprised if they moved back in the direction of fostering independence and resilience in their own children, which they were often denied themselves ("I'm not hoping to let my kids spend hours on their phone the way my parent let me").

Again, I am not advocating that we as parents go back to another era, but I do feel the pendulum has swung much too far in the other direction, which likely plays an important role in the decline in children's mental health.

We will revisit the topic of independence later in the book, when we shift our attention to treatment.

What Does This All Mean?

Why all of this depression, anxiety, and self-harm among children and teenagers? And why now? Let me attempt to bring together all these disparate pieces of information and research, along with my own clinical observations of working with adolescents, and paint the clinical big picture.

The most compelling clue so far for the explosion in mental health challenges among children and teens is that it coincides with the onset of their regular use of smartphones. Beginning in 2004, the Pew Internet & American Life Project began collecting data on the percentage of adolescents ages 12 to 17 who had their own smartphones and found that the percentage rose very rapidly. In 2004 it was 45%; in 2006 it had risen to 63%; in 2008 to 71%; and by 2018 that number jumped to pretty much all teenagers (95%) (Lenhart, 2009). In my practice, I don't know of a single teenager who doesn't have a phone (unless of course it was temporarily taken away from them for some misdeed). My youngest client to get a cellphone was seven years old (sadly, a gift from Grandma).

In her excellent book, *iGen: Why Today's Super-Connected Kids Are Growing Up Less Rebellious, More Tolerant, Less Happy—and Completely Unprepared for Adulthood—and What That Means for the Rest of Us*, psychologist Jean Twenge outlines the relevant research indicating the relationship between smartphone use and the increase in child and adolescent mental illness (Twenge, 2017). (Twenge uses the term iGen but Gen Z is more commonly used for children born between 1995 and 2012.) The uptick in mental health challenges appears to have coincided with the year 2012, which is right about the time a majority of people started using smartphones. That smartphones and other devices have changed our lives in extraordinary ways is undeniable, and their impact on our children's well-being is now starting to become clear.

I know, I know. Adults always tell kids that they spend too much time on their phones and it's not good for them, which drives them crazy. But that's the truth—they do spend too much time on them. Remember, we learned that by their own admission, nearly half of teens say they are addicted to their phones and nearly that same percentage acknowledge being on their phone "almost constantly" (up to nine hours a day).

And for most kids that's likely not a problem. If a child is psychologically healthy, not necessarily prone to depression or anxiety (we'll look at temperamental differences in Chapter 5), have a family life that is generally peaceful, loving, and low-stress, with a solid, positive friend group, that kid is likely going to be okay if they spend a lot of time of their phone. But these are not the kids I see in my practice. Far from it.

Here's what I see more typically. Children and teens spend *inordinate* amounts of time on devices. Remember, we also learned that there is a correlation between time on devices and increased mental health problems—a dose-related effect—more depressed, more anxious, and more suicidal. So, the number of hours per day on the phone all by itself can be a risk factor or vulnerability for the onset of a mental health disorder. Remember too, that excessive time on a device also creates a time imbalance (the crowding-out effect). Less time with family, less time for other, healthier, activities like exercise, sports, or time outside, or perhaps even more important—enough sleep. The importance of adequate sleep for mood regulation cannot be overstated. (Ask yourself what kind of a mood you're in after a few nights of not sleeping well. Now multiply that by weeks on end.) More time on a device also means more time for unfavorably comparing oneself with others on social media ("There must be something wrong with me. No one wants to hang out with me") and more opportunities to be bullied or harassed. We also learned from the research on COVID that simply being parked in a bedroom, mostly alone, and rarely leaving the house is also a vulnerability for depression.

Many of the kids I work with are desperately lonely. COVID set the stage for that for many of them, but there are quite a few others that weren't great in the friends department before the pandemic. They struggled to make and keep friends, which I believe becomes more difficult as kids get older (and more difficult for adults too, by the way). In truth, we all want connection—it's wired into us as social primates. To be a part of a group, to feel like we belong and are wanted is a basic, fundamental human need for most of us. These kids spend time on their phones often *because* they have no friends and want to connect with someone, anyone that will talk to them.

But who are these people with whom they've connected? Pretty much every kid (and sometimes adults) that you would never want your child or teenager to be talking to. Many of them are also equally lonely kids struggling with their own mental health issues. This, in part, is where social contagion theory becomes highly relevant. Recall that when people interact with other people who are depressed, they are far more likely to become depressed themselves. This is also true with substance use, anxiety, and self-harm. So, a lonely, depressed, and sometimes suicidal teen regularly interacting with other lonely, depressed, and sometimes suicidal teens is a recipe for big problems.

Smartphones also open the door for a struggling adolescent to communicate with not just a few equally struggling teens but with entire communities of them. There are numerous virtual communities comprised of depressed, lonely, and self-harming kids. I find Discord to be the biggest offender, with multiple "servers" (chat rooms) of equally disaffected, unhappy youth, although I'm certain there are other platforms of which I am not aware that offer the same, and many others in development. Teenagers get drawn into these "echo chambers" of despair and mutually reinforce each other's dysfunction. Think of it as a psychological race to the bottom.

Many of the teenagers I work with are also very closed off and disconnected from their parents. They essentially go quiet, which means that whatever they're seeing or learning about online, they have to make sense of all on their own. They no longer can turn to the very people best positioned to help guide them or give them good advice. Cell phones do not care about our children—their developers care only about kids buying more of them and keeping them glued to the device to generate advertising dollars.

I find that just about all parents are concerned about how much time their child spends in their bedroom on a device. That it's a problem is obvious to them. But in most cases, in my experience, parents do minimal to no monitoring of their teenagers' devices. Parents generally don't understand the technology very well (kids are way better at it) and vastly underestimate the harm the devices are causing. I tell parents that time on a device is like a slow intravenous (IV) drip going into their child's arm. Parents generally want to pull out the IV but here's the problem—just about all kids resist this heavily. It leads to massive, heated arguments, and many kids will throw down the gauntlet: "If you take my phone I'm going to kill myself." Much more on how to respond to this later.

In order to really understand what's happening to our kids' mental health we need to extend social contagion theory even further. I believe so many kids are depressed, anxious, and suicidal now not just because they're being bullied, or are scared someone will come and shoot up the school, but because we live in a present-day culture in which depression, anxiety, and suicide are all talked about constantly—on the news, social media, and in the classroom. Kids cut themselves because other kids cut themselves. Every kid knows other kids who do it, and so in their minds, it's an option. And the prevailing, popular notion discussed freely among teenagers is that self-harm *makes you feel better*. In truth, most of my patients eventually come to acknowledge that it doesn't actually do that; it's a myth. In reality, over time, it makes them feel much worse, but I bet they don't hear that very often on Instagram or TikTok.

So, yes, our children and teens are more depressed, anxious, and suicidal than they have ever been. But the reasons for this are multifaceted and complicated, making treatment equally complicated. For example, take a teenager who presents for therapy with depressed mood and self-harm. A straightforward approach to their treatment might include starting them on an antidepressant and some traditional cognitive behavioral therapy, or maybe dialectical therapy (more on these later). The therapist would probably help teach some mood regulation skills, discuss the importance of spending less time on their phone, maybe setting aside the phone earlier, getting more sleep, and so on. They might also talk about the value of doing chores around the house or getting their driver's license.

All useful stuff to be sure. But my goodness, look at what all these approaches leave out of the equation. What about social contagion—what role is it playing in the child's life? Who do they know that's cutting? What does their friend group look like and how do you change it for the better? Putting their phone down and getting more sleep is a great idea but what kid can actually do that on their own? Telling parents to invite kids out of their bedrooms is a great idea but how do you handle it if they won't? How can an antidepressant change who a kid is talking to at 3:00 a.m.? And what teenager will voluntarily start doing chores without their parents making that happen?

And how can one therapist possibly have an impact on all of these complex systems just by seeing the kid one time per week?

This book is about adding an awful lot more horsepower to the therapeutic engine. Each of the negative influences discussed in this and the previous chapter must be assessed, parsed out, and ultimately *disrupted* in ways that are beneficial to the child or adolescent. To do the job right, I'm going to need some powerful allies who can change the larger social situation in ways that one therapist, in many cases, simply cannot.

And I think I know exactly who those allies are.

Chief Takeaways from Chapter 2

For Parents
- Your child's mental health is susceptible to the effects of social contagion, an aspect of human nature in which our moods and behaviors are highly influenced by the moods and behaviors of others.
- When your child or teen is regularly interacting with a peer who is depressed, anxious, or suicidal, it increases the likelihood of your child being that way too.
- Even as little as a 20-minute interaction between your child and someone who is depressed increases the risk of your child feeling depressed as well.
- Try to learn more about your child's friends (or anyone with whom they regularly interact). If they are connected with a kid with similar mental health problems, that is likely going to make your child's problems worse by creating an "echo chamber," a mutual worsening of each other's symptoms. (We'll talk later about what to do if this is the case.)
- You can help your child become more resilient, an essential life skill, by asking them to engage in age-appropriate responsibilities such as doing chores, getting their driver's license, and getting a part-time job. Try to let them make their own decisions when appropriate so they can learn from their mistakes and tolerate the discomfort this brings.

For Clinicians
- One of the most important things you can do to help your patients is to learn everything you can about their friends.
- Provide psychoeducation on the fact that emotions and behaviors are socially contagious—some degree of your patient's low mood can be attributed just to whomever they're talking to and whether that person is struggling with similar issues.
- When trying to understand a child's symptoms, consider whether there might be a "functional" aspect to them, i.e., something the symptoms do for the child that gives them an incentive not to let go of them (more on this later).
- Many Gen Z kids are slower to grow up and do not become resilient because they are not engaging in age-typical independent tasks. Encourage your patients to do so and then identify and remove any barriers preventing this from occurring.
- Remember, parents have a much greater ability to reduce screen time than you do. Make use of them and work to vastly reduce time spent on devices.

References

Arendt, F., Scherr, S., & Romer, D. (2019). Effects of exposure to self-harm on social media: Evidence from a two-wave panel study among young adults. *New Media & Society, 21*(11–12), 2422–2442. 10.1177/1461444819850106

Baker, T. G., & Lewis, S. P. (2013). Responses to online photographs of non-suicidal self-injury: A thematic analysis. *Archives of Suicide Research, 17*(3), 223–235. 10.1080/13811118.2013.805642

Bazrafshan, M.-R., Sharif, F., Molazem, Z., & Mani, A. (2016). Exploring the risk factors contributing to suicide attempt among adolescents: A qualitative study. *Iranian Journal of Nursing and Midwifery Research, 21*(1), 93–99. 10.4103 %2F1735-9066.174747

Blumer, H. (1939). Collective behavior. In R. E. Park (Ed.), *Principles of sociology* (pp. 219–288). Barnes & Noble.

Brown, R. C., Fischer, T., Goldwich, A. D., Keller, F., Young, R., & Plener, P. L. (2018). #cutting: Non-suicidal self-injury (NSSI) on Instagram. *Psychological Medicine, 48*(2), 337–346. 10.1017/s0033291717001751

Cacioppo, J. T., Fowler, J. H., & Christakis, N. A. (2009). Alone in the crowd: The structure and spread of loneliness in a large social network. *Journal of Personality and Social Psychology, 97*(6), 977–991. 10.1037/a0016076

Cheng, A. T. A., Hawton, K., Chen, T. H. H., Yen, A. M. F., Chang, J.-C., Chong, M.-Y., Liu, C.-Y., Lee, Y., Teng, P.-R., & Chen, L.-C. (2007). The influence of media reporting of a celebrity suicide on suicidal behavior in patients with a history of depressive disorder. *Journal of Affective Disorders, 103*(1–3), 69–75. 10.1016/j.jad.2007.01.021

Christakis, N. A., & Fowler, J. H. (2007). The spread of obesity in a large social network over 32 years. *The New England Journal of Medicine, 357*(4), 370–379. 10.1056/nejmsa066082

Cline, F., & Fay, J. (1990). *Parenting with love and logic: Teaching children responsibility*. Pinon Press.

Duffin, E. (2023). *U.S. teens (16–19) who are enrolled in school and working 1985–2021*. Statista. https://www.statista.com/statistics/477668/percentage-of-youth-who-are-enrolled-in-school-and-working-in-the-us/

Federal Highway Administration. (2020, February 28). *Distribution of licensed drivers – 2018: By sex and percentage in each age group and relation to population*. https://www.fhwa.dot.gov/policyinformation/statistics/2018/dl20.cfm

Florsheim, L. (2023, March 30). Sleepovers are now a battleground. *The Wall Street Journal*. https://www.wsj.com/articles/sleepovers-divide-parents-allow-or-not-d9b8072c

Gladwell, M. (2006). *The tipping point: How little things can make a big difference*. Little, Brown and Company.

Gould, M. S. (2001). Suicide and the media. *Annals of the New York Academy of Sciences, 932*(1), 200–224. 10.1111/j.1749-6632.2001.tb05807.x

Gould, M. S., & Lake, A. M. (2013). The contagion of suicidal behavior. In *Contagion of violence: Workshop summary* (pp. 68–73). The National Academies Press. 10.17226/13489

Gould, M. S., Wallenstein, S., Kleinman, M. H., O'Carroll, P., & Mercy, J. (1990). Suicide clusters: An examination of age-specific effects. *American Journal of Public Health, 80*(2): 211–212. 10.2105/ajph.80.2.211

Gould, M. S., Kleinman, M. H., Lake, A. M., Forman, J., & Midle, J. B. (2014). Newspaper coverage of suicide and initiation of suicide clusters in teenagers in the USA, 1988-96: A retrospective, population-based, case-control study. *The Lancet Psychiatry, 1*(1), 34–43. 10.1016/s2215-0366(14)70225-1

Gould, M. S., Lake, A. M., Kleinman, M., Galfalvy, H., Chowdhury, S., & Madnick, A. (2018). Exposure to suicide in high schools: Impact on serious suicidal ideation/behavior, depression, maladaptive coping strategies, and attitudes toward help-seeking. *International Journal of Environmental Research and Public Health, 15*(3), 455. 10.3390/ijerph15030455

Gray, P., Lancy, D. F., & Bjorklund, D. F. (2023). Decline in independent activity as a cause of decline in children's mental well-being: Summary of the evidence. *The Journal of Pediatrics.* 10.1016/j.jpeds.2023.02.004

Hammen, C., Burge, D., & Adrian, C. (1991). Timing of mother and child depression in a longitudinal study of children at risk. *Journal of Consulting and Clinical Psychology, 59*(2), 341–345. 10.1037/0022-006X.59.2.341

Hatfield, E., Cacioppo, J. T., & Rapson, R. L. (1993). Emotional contagion. *Current Directions in Psychological Science, 2*(3), 96–99. 10.1111/1467-8721.ep10770953

Hatfield, E., Carpenter, M., & Rapson, R. L. (2014). Emotional contagion as a precursor to collective emotions. In C. von Scheve & M. Salmela (Eds.), *Collective emotions: Perspectives from psychology, philosophy, and sociology* (pp. 108–122). Oxford University Press. 10.1093/acprof:oso/9780199659180.003.0008

Heyman, I., Liang, H., & Hedderly, T. (2021). COVID-19 related increase in childhood tics and tic-like attacks. *Archives of Disease in Childhood, 106*, 420–421. 10.1136/archdischild-2021-321748

Hogue, A., & Steinberg, L. (1995). Homophily of internalized distress in adolescent peer groups. *Developmental Psychology, 31*(6), 897–906. 10.1037/0012-1649.31.6.897

Hunley, S. (2017, January 10). *Helicopter parenting: Can it cause anxiety?* Anxiety.org. https://www.anxiety.org/helicopter-parenting-associated-with-anxiety-in-young-adults

Jarvi, S., Jackson, B., Swenson, L., & Crawford, H. (2013). The impact of social contagion on non-suicidal self-injury: A review of the literature. *Archives of Suicide Research, 17*(1), 1–19. 10.1080/13811118.2013.748404

Joiner, T. E., Jr. (1994). Contagious depression: Existence, specificity to depressed symptoms, and the role of reassurance seeking. *Journal of Personality and Social Psychology, 67*(2), 287–296. 10.1037/0022-3514.67.2.287

Joiner, T. E., Jr. (1999). The clustering and contagion of suicide. *Current Directions in Psychological Science, 8*(3), 89–92. 10.1111/1467-8721.00021

Jones, T. F., Craig, A. S., Hoy, D., Gunter, E. W., Ashley, D. L., Barr, D. B., Brock, J. W., & Schaffner, W. (2000). Mass psychogenic illness attributed to toxic exposure at a high school. *The New England Journal of Medicine, 342*(2), 96–100. 10.1056/nejm200001133420206

Katz, J., Beach, S. R. H., & Joiner, T. E., Jr. (1999). Contagious depression in dating couples. *Journal of Social and Clinical Psychology, 18*(1), 1–13. 10.1521/jscp.1999.18.1.1

Kharabsheh, S., Al-Otoum, H., Clements, J., Abbas, A., Khuri-Bulos, N., Belbesi, A., Gaafar, T., & Dellepiane, N. (2001). Mass psychogenic illness following tetanus-diphtheria toxoid vaccination in Jordan. *Bulletin of the World Health Organization, 79*(8), 764–770.

Le Bon, G. (1896). *The crowd: A study of the popular mind* (T. Fisher Unwin, Trans.). T. Fisher Unwin (Original work published 1895).

Lenhart, A. (2009). *Teens and mobile phones over the past five years: Pew Internet looks back.* Pew Research Center. https://www.pewresearch.org/internet/2009/08/19/teens-and-mobile-phones-over-the-past-five-years-pew-internet-looks-back/

Locher, D. A. (2002). *Collective behavior.* Prentice Hall.

Love, H., May, R.W., Cui, M., & Fincham, F. D. (2019). Helicopter parenting, self-control, and school burnout among emerging adults. *Journal of Child and Family Studies, 29*, 327–337. 10.1007/s10826-019-01560-z

Lowe, E. D. (2019). Social change and Micronesian suicide mortality: A test of competing hypotheses. *Cross-Cultural Research, 53*(1), 3–32. 10.1177/1069397118759004

Luebbe, A. M., Mancini, K. J., Kiel, E. J., Spangler, B. R., Semlak, J. L., & Fussner, L. M. (2018). Dimensionality of helicopter parenting and relations to emotional, decision-making, and academic functioning in emerging adults. *Assessment, 25*(7), 841–857. 10.1177/1073191116665907

Mednick, S. C., Christakis, N. A., & Fowler, J. H. (2010). The spread of sleep loss influences drug use in adolescent social networks. *PLoS One, 5*(3), Article e9775. 10.1371/journal.pone.0009775

Montgomery, N. (2010, May). *The negative impact of helicopter parenting on personality* [Poster presentation]. Association of Psychological Science, Boston, MA, United States.

Murray, C. D., & Fox, J. (2006). Do internet self-harm discussion groups alleviate or exacerbate self-harming behaviour? *Australian e-journal for the Advancement of Mental Health, 5*(3), 225–233. 10.5172/jamh.5.3.225

National Center for Injury Prevention and Control. (n.d.). *Suicide, suicide attempt, or self-harm clusters.* U.S. Department of Health and Human Services, Centers for Disease Control and Prevention. https://www.cdc.gov/suicide/resources/suicide-clusters.html

Niederkrotenthaler, T., Braun, M., Pirkis, J., Till, B., Stack, S., Sinyor, M., Tran, U. S., Voracek, M., Cheng, Q., Arendt, F., Scherr, S., Yip, P. S. F., & Spittal, M. J. (2020). Association between suicide reporting in the media and suicide: Systematic review and meta-analysis. *British Medical Journal, 368*, Article m575. 10.1136/bmj.m575

Nock, M. K., & Prinstein, M. J. (2004). A functional approach to the assessment of self-mutilative behavior. *Journal of Consulting and Clinical Psychology, 72*(5), 885–890. 10.1037/0022-006x.72.5.885

O'Sullivan, S. (2021). *The sleeping beauties: And other stories of mystery illness.* Pantheon.

Papadima, M. (2019). Rethinking self-harm: A psychoanalytic consideration of hysteria and social contagion. *Journal of Child Psychotherapy, 45*(3), 291–307. 10.1080/0075417X.2019.1700297

Perlmutter, L. (2023, June). Was mass hysteria behind the mysterious case of 227 middle school students fainting last fall? *Insider: Science.* https://www. businessinsider.com/was-mass-hysteria-behind-a-mysterious-middle-school-fainting-epidemic-2023-6

Poijula, S., Wahlberg, K. E., & Dyregrov, A. (2001). Adolescent suicide and suicide contagion in three secondary schools. *International Journal of Emergency Mental Health, 3*(3), 163–168.

Purington, A., & Whitlock, J. (2010, February). Non-suicidal self-injury in the media. *The Prevention Researcher, 17*(1), 11–14.

Romer, D., Jamieson, P. E., & Jamieson, K. H. (2006). Are news reports of suicide contagious? A stringent test in six U.S. cities. *Journal of Communication, 56*(2), 253–270. 10.1111/j.1460-2466.2006.00018.x

Rosenquist, J. N., Murabito, J., Fowler, J. H., & Christakis, N. A. (2010). The spread of alcohol consumption behavior in a large social network. *Annals of Internal Medicine, 52*(7), 426–433. 10.7326/0003-4819-152-7-201004060-00007

Schwartz, S. (2018, August 15). Helicopter parenting: From good intentions to poor outcomes. *The Gottman Institute.* https://www.gottman.com/blog/helicopter-parenting-good-intentions-poor-outcomes/

Schwartz-Mette, R. A., & Rose, A. J. (2012). Co-rumination mediates contagion of internalizing symptoms within youths' friendships. *Developmental Psychology, 48*(5), 1355–1365. 10.1037/a0027484

Segrin, C., & Dillard, J. P. (1992). The interactional theory of depression: A meta-analysis of the research literature. *Journal of Social and Clinical Psychology, 11*(1), 43–70. 10.1521/jscp.1992.11.1.43

Serra Poirier, C., Brendgen, M., Vitaro, F., Dionne, G., & Boivin, M. (2017). Contagion of anxiety symptoms among adolescent siblings: A twin study. *Journal of Research on Adolescence, 27*(1), 65–77. 10.1111/jora.12254

Shaw, P. V., Wilson, G. A., & Antony, M. M. (2021). Examination of emotional contagion and social anxiety using novel video stimuli. *Anxiety, Stress, & Coping, 34*(2), 215–227. 10.1080/10615806.2020.1839729

Srivastav, D., & Lal Mathur, M. N. (2021). Helicopter parenting and adolescent development: From the perspective of mental health. In L. Benedetto & M. Ingrassia (Eds.), *Parenting—Studies by an ecocultural and transactional perspective* (pp. 71–89). IntechOpen. 10.5772/intechopen.83010

Stack, S. (2005). Suicide in the media: A quantitative review of studies based on non-fictional stories. *Suicide and Life-Threatening Behavior, 35*(2), 121–133. 10.1521/suli.35.2.121.62877

Stevens, E. A., & Prinstein, M. J. (2005). Peer contagion of depressogenic attributional styles among adolescents: A longitudinal study. *Journal of Abnormal Child Psychology, 33*(1), 25–37. 10.1007/s10802-005-0931-2

Strack, S., & Coyne, J. C. (1983). Social confirmation of dysphoria: Shared and private reactions to depression. *Journal of Personality and Social Psychology, 44*(4), 798–806. 10.1037/0022-3514.44.4.798

Twaddle, I. K. B., Hezel, F. X., Rubinstein, D. H., Arriola, J. E. H., David, A. M., Nena, H. J., Meno, C. G., Mauricio, A. D., Anefal, J. B., Thomson, M. A., Temengil, E. J., Palemar, I. L., Tafledep, H., Maipi, I. L., & Wasson, V. H. (2022). Psychology in Micronesia. In G. J. Rich & N. A. Ramkumar (Eds.), *Psychology in Oceania and the Caribbean* (1st ed., pp. 3–17). Springer. 10. 1007/978-3-030-87763-7

Twenge, J. M. (2017). *iGen: Why today's super-connected kids are growing up less rebellious, more tolerant, less happy—and completely unprepared for adulthood—and what that means for the rest of us.* Atria Books.

Wallace, J. B. (2015, March 13). Why children need chores. *The Wall Street Journal.* https://www.wsj.com/articles/why-children-need-chores-1426262655

Walters, M. (2022). *How your mental health might be 'syncing up' with your partner's.* Stylist. https://www.stylist.co.uk/relationships/dating-love/mental-health-syncing-up-with-partner-study/690569

3 Righting the Ship
Getting Families Back on Course

It is common at the outset of treatment for families with a child or adolescent with a mental health condition to have drifted very far off course. This typically happens slowly and by degrees due to a combination of the child's temperament (more on this in the next chapter), the severity of the child's presenting problems, and what are usually powerful social and situational influences. Family life with a self-harming, suicidal, anxious, or very oppositional child or adolescent often in no way resembles how parents had envisioned family life.

Things are not right and everyone knows it.

The resulting effect is an incredible amount of pain, loss, and upset. With a self-harming or highly anxious child, parents are understandably careful to avoid causing them any kind of stress that might lead to conflict, or perhaps yet another upset or crisis. Similarly, with a highly oppositional and explosive child or teen, parents work very hard not to make them angry. Parents and siblings are walking on eggshells constantly. This invariably leads to giving in to what the child wants—more time on devices, odd sleeping patterns, less time out of their bedrooms, less time with friends, or falling far behind in school (or worse, dropping out altogether). Most therapists who see just the child individually are often at a loss as to how to help, and, in fact, in many instances, they advise parents not to ask anything of their children to avoid stressing them even further.

I worked with a boy who had just been discharged from a psychiatric hospital, and the instructions his parents were given were to lower his stress by allowing him to play video games as a "self-soothe skill." As you might imagine, the boy wholeheartedly endorsed this idea (what kid wouldn't?) and when his parents asked him to consider cutting back on his gaming time, he reminded them that they were told it was therapeutic for him.

While it makes sense to temporarily reduce stress for a depressed teen who has experienced some sort of mental health crisis or to try to avoid angering someone prone to irritability, maintaining lowered expectations

DOI: 10.4324/9781003397366-5

is not sustainable, resulting in an inevitable stalemate that can be highly stressful for families and not at all helpful for kids.

Here's how it often plays out, in my experience.

For a variety of reasons that we will explore throughout this book, a child begins to go off track from what was previously a reasonably decent level of functioning to something far from that. Maybe the social isolation from the pandemic began to take its toll and the child started to become lonely and feel down. Or maybe something is happening in their friend group that is upsetting to them—they've been ostracized or singled out and tormented by cyberbullying on social media. Maybe they've been spending too much time on their phone in general (which, as we've learned, worsens depression) or maybe they've connected virtually with one or more less-than-ideal peers who themselves are struggling (or worse, adults claiming to be peers). Perhaps they just started middle or high school and the academic demands have increased such that they're falling far behind for the first time. Something could be going on at home; for example, increased family conflict due to economic stressors, or parents fighting and perhaps on the brink of divorce. Anything, really—just something that creates a vulnerability in the child.

This initial vulnerability might then result in the child engaging in unhelpful coping strategies and attempts to feel better that don't work— more time on their phone or other devices and more time in their bedrooms. This, in turn, leads to a cascade of other problems, such as communicating with peers who, at best, might be struggling themselves or, at worst, tell the child that their parents are to blame for their unhappiness. Interacting with other depressed, anxious, or suicidal teens sets the stage for emotional and behavioral contagion, and repeated exposure to dysphoric conversations and negative social media content, such as watching awful TikTok videos of other unhappy, suicidal kids in darkened bedrooms, creating the illusion that "everyone feels this way." Seeing other kids on social media also struggling with depression or anxiety provides what is known as "social proof," a term coined by Robert Cialdini to describe the tendency for people to copy the actions of others when they're not sure of how to behave in a particular situation (Cialdini, 2009). The child becomes more withdrawn from the family, refusing to leave their bedroom and becoming more closed off and less communicative. Depressed and/or anxious moods become predominant, often coupled with hostility toward their parents.

At this point, parents are becoming increasingly confused and scared. The child isn't saying much at all, and when parents ask what's going on, most kids respond by giving a very unsatisfying answer: "I don't know" (or, I suppose, the even worse "Leave me alone"). This may be frustrating for parents to hear but I do believe it's an honest answer. The child knows they are unhappy, but they can't put into words why. That's because they really don't know. They simply do not have an awareness of, or an understanding about, how all of these situational variables are affecting their well-being—isolating in their bedrooms, pulling away from family, excessive time on devices doing God knows what, and so on. So, the explanation they give for what's making them unhappy often doesn't make sense because it's based on very unreliable data.

As such, the child begins to gradually withdraw from the world and function more and more poorly. Less interacting with family, not wanting to leave the house or go anywhere, pulling away from friends (if friends are even still in the picture), often refusing to take care of their basic hygiene such as showering or brushing their teeth, not doing much homework or no homework at all, falling behind in school or refusing to go altogether, not wanting to help out around the house as they might have previously, not pursuing their driver's license or a job—just the basics of living in which we would reasonably expect most kids to engage. And, obviously, not all kids fit this precise pattern or exhibit exactly these behaviors, but these are the most common I have seen routinely in my practice.

"Wonky" Patterns of Reinforcement

Real trouble begins when parents start to recognize that they've gotten themselves into a mess and, at some point, they try to set some reasonable limits again ("You have to go to school!"). Usually, this begins by having endless conversations about why the kid shouldn't spend so much time on their phones, but ultimately these conversations most often go exactly nowhere. Next, they might ask the child directly to spend less time on their phones or gaming, which most kids usually agree to but then don't actually do. If parents start to push things, like doing homework, taking showers, doing chores, or trying to make them come out of their rooms more often, this often leads to serious conflict. Ultimately, some parents might then try to restrict time on devices or take them away altogether but, my goodness, that can go *very* badly. Now it's a massive conflict, and kids defend their device use or time in their room with a vengeance.

These are the most common things kids will tell their parents when they try to set limits (if you are a parent, I bet these will sound very familiar to you):

> *"Being on my phone is the only thing that makes me less depressed."*
> *"Why are you taking things from me that are the only things I still enjoy? Don't you understand that makes me feel worse?"*
> *"Now you're not letting me talk to my friends? I thought I was supposed to be social?"*

"Why are you always talking about school? You care more about school than you do my mental health. See, you don't care about me!"
"I can't help out around the house because I'm too depressed."
"I can't do school right until I'm feeling less anxious."
"My phone (or friends) keeps me from cutting. It would be worse if I did that right?"
"Talking with my friends is my coping skill."

And here's the real showstopper:

"If you try and take my phone I'm going to kill myself."

When that last card is thrown down, watch out. No parent, under any circumstances, is going to push after that, and if they hadn't backed off from expectations completely before then they almost certainly will now.

And then what? They ask for less and less and the child's depression and anxiety gets worse and worse. Time in their bedroom increases, they fall further behind in school, time spent online with others increases, and so on.

And the child or teen becomes massively reinforced for saying they're going to kill themself. And it works: parents back off and ask nothing of them.

[*Note: a quick introduction to the concept of reinforcement because it's very important when it comes to understanding, and ultimately changing, a child's behavior. Simply put, a behavior is positively reinforced (made stronger) when something follows the behavior that makes it more likely that behavior will occur again in the future. There are a million real-world examples of this (like giving your dog a treat when it sits, a bonus at work for a productive year, a gold star at the top of a child's homework, and so on)*]

If the child says, "Give me back my phone or I'm going to kill myself" and the phone is returned, the threat of suicide has been massively reinforced. A child doesn't need to know on a conscious level that their behavior has just been reinforced—often this happens without their awareness—but reinforced it is and so similar statements will very likely occur again. All human beings—in fact almost all animals—respond to reinforcement. The return of the phone also incorrectly reinforces the parents' behavior, in that the kid is now less upset and the crisis of the moment (and the parents' fears) has been relieved (something that goes by the very confusing name of "negative reinforcement"). The kid gets upset and parents give in—a mutual but wonky (unhelpful) reinforcement pattern that keeps dysfunctional behavior locked firmly into place.

Please note that I have no judgment whatsoever for both the parents and the kid for finding themselves in this situation. The process just unfolds under the right set of conditions without anyone's awareness, and, when it does, it's very hard for the family to get back on course without some professional assistance.

I think what is influencing the child's withdrawal from the world is fueled at least in part by what is known about how human beings are wired to take the path of least resistance, due to what is referred to as the Principle of Least Effort. Nobuhiro Hagura, at the Institute of Cognitive Neuroscience, University College London, conducted a study in which participants took part in a series of tests where they had to judge whether a cloud of dots on a screen was moving to the left or to the right (Hagura et al., 2017). Once they had made their decision, they moved a handle held in their left or right hand respectively. Next, a load was gradually added to one of the handles, which made it more difficult to move. Interestingly, the subjects' perceptions as to what they were seeing became biased (the movement of the clouds), and they started to avoid the effortful response. For example, if the weight was added to the left handle, they were more likely to judge the dots to be moving to the right. That decision was slightly easier for them to express, all of which was occurring unconsciously. Think about this: when choosing a particular course of action, we are all biased to select the least effortful option. For example, if my car breaks down, I'm going to come up with a ride that's the easiest for me to obtain—I'll call a tow truck, or ask my wife to come pick me up, and so on, but I'd never just walk home unless an easier option was unavailable.

Depressed children and teenagers do exactly the same thing. I've no doubt that the longer someone disengages from a fairly typical teenage activity, such as interacting with family members, doing homework, going to school, spending time involving anything other than a device, etc. the harder it becomes for them to start doing it again. Doing so, at least to them perceptually, is going to feel like effort, and if parents inadvertently reinforce avoidant behavior, it is easy to see why the child or teen's level of functioning declines over time. This is just what people do.

We should probably also talk about the role that power imbalances play in all of this. It probably doesn't come as a surprise to you when I say kids have very little power in a family system. They're basically told what to do and the general expectation is that they mostly do it. This is especially true for younger children; we tell them what to do all the time. While kids might not always do as we ask (far from it), it's usually understood that parents do get to tell them what to do and that's how the family universe works. Tantrum if you want because it's your bedtime, but, you're going to go to bed eventually, and we all know it.

As kids get older, the notion of autonomy and wanting to be independent grows gradually stronger the further into adolescence they get. Kids become much more aware of, and increasingly less tolerant of, their parents (and others) telling them what to do, so they look for opportunities to claim some of that power. This can take a variety of forms, such as being slow to do a chore when asked (many times they'll do it, but only when they feel like it), coming home a little past curfew just because, and so on. Communication patterns can change as well, in ways that are about power: some kids start to curse at their parents or generally speak disrespectfully to them, yell at them when angry, or repeatedly interrupt them in a conversation or argument. These are all just indications of a human being wanting more autonomy and trying to level out the power differential.

So if the child's mood is low, and if everything seems like an effort, they, like most, will choose the path of least effort. If they make a threatening comment ("If I can't be on my phone then I'm going to cut myself"), the teen quickly learns that, oh my goodness, now the power differential has massively shifted. *This works. Now I can do what I want, which is WAY better than being told what to do.* And here is what parents say about this power shift: "I feel like I have no authority anymore. I used to be able to ask them to do things, but I feel like now I can't."

Again, I don't judge kids for any of this. We all want power, especially when we're not accustomed to having it. And when we get a taste of it, we will go to great lengths to hang on to it. But here's the thing. As much as kids like having some of that power, they're still kids and often don't have the wisdom, maturity, or life experience to make sound decisions. Failing all of their classes is the path of least effort, and the kid will give you ten "good" reasons why they're not going to school. But the decision to drop out of school at the age of 15 is most definitely not a sound one and should not be left to them.

One of the most difficult, but important, parts of treatment is restoring a fairly natural power structure that's been absent since the onset of the mental health condition. Gently, slowly, respectfully, but getting kids back into the world and giving parents the chance to parent again is essential. And I'm convinced too that when kids finally relinquish that power back over to their parents they actually feel much better and their general mood improves.

Let's go back to our phone example. Instead of returning it to the teen after a threat of suicide, what if the parent sticks to their guns and doesn't return the phone? But what happens if the child then makes good on what they said and cuts themselves? Or ends up in the emergency room because they are having suicidal thoughts? *Uh oh.* At this point, understandably, the parents are probably going to return the damn phone. Who wouldn't do that? Surely trying to get the child off their phone and out of their bedroom isn't worth the risk of another self-harm event? But the self-harm has just been massively reinforced. In fact, if the parent were to acquiesce and give the phone back after holding out a bit, then the reinforcement pattern was made much worse. As a result of that interaction, the child was given further incentive to level up on the threat (carrying it out), which gives the parents further incentive to back off and give in.

Herein lies the complexity of my work.

Children and teens who are highly oppositional and even aggressive essentially follow this same already entrenched, unhelpful pattern of reinforcement. These kids often "light up" when asked to do something they don't want to do (homework, helping around the house, getting off a device, being respectful, etc.). They get really angry and often yell and curse at their parents, and in some cases damage property or become physically aggressive. If you think about it, it's a pretty effective strategy to get parents to stop asking things of them ("Why bother? It's not worth the fight") and for the kid to avoid any task or request made of them. Who wants some massive explosion? Again, it's not that oppositional kids have consciously adopted this strategy—they've just been reinforced over and over again for blowing up without any awareness of this whatsoever, so of course they're just going to keep doing it.

In my experience, many of the more extreme behaviors exhibited by kids with mental health challenges are less about their mental health condition and more about the function these behaviors serve, including kids who self-harm or are explosive. When a kid gets what they want—such as not being held accountable, or avoiding things they don't want to do—by yelling at their parents or threatening suicide, that behavior serves a function. Is it fair to say that because of those behaviors the child then gets labeled with a "mental health condition"? I don't think so. For example, we often say a teen isn't doing their homework because they are depressed, which in some cases is obviously true, but, in most cases, the child's behavior brings something of value to them. Assessing the function of a given behavior is an important part of treatment because if we know a behavior has a function, we can intervene in a variety of ways to change that situational influence.

This is usually the point at which families first present for treatment. Everything has ground to a halt—the child or teen is highly depressed (looks depressed, sounds depressed, says they're depressed, etc.), spends almost every waking moment on a device, rarely leaves their room, stays up all night and sleeps very late into the day, communicating mostly with other depressed or anxious kids, contemplating suicide, and becoming disconnected from and often hostile toward their parents. Parents, on their side of it, feel terrified and helpless, waiting for the next bad thing to happen, and often feel angry and resentful that they can no longer parent their child or set limits in any reasonable way.

All of this must be disrupted over the course of treatment. And all through this book I'm going to show you how to do exactly that.

The general belief, both lay and professional, is that a child will resume a normal life once they start feeling better. While this is probably true in some cases, in my work I find it to be the reverse—children and teens start to feel better when they begin the process of stepping back into life with the support of their parents and the treatment team.

Kids feel better when they do better, not the other way around.

Reversing the course on this is challenging for both clinicians and families but in my work I have found this to be vital in treating serious child and adolescent mental illness. This is consistent with what we know about the treatment of depression, which, as far as I am aware, does not include telling patients that they should spend more time in a darkened bedroom. We do not sit back and wait for the child to feel better before asking more of them; we start asking more of them on week one.

And we're relentless in this pursuit. Safely, of course, and balanced with an enormous amount of kindness and compassion, gentleness, playfulness, and affection. We never give up asking kids and their parents for change, but we do it slowly and, hopefully, in the nicest way possible.

The Gentle Ask

So, change results by doing, not avoiding. In Intensive Family-Focused Therapy (IFFT), we begin by using what we call the "gentle-ask" strategy, whereby some relatively low-stakes behavior is targeted for change right away: showering once a day, for example, or completing one chore day. I think of this as low-hanging fruit, targeting a new behavior that I don't think is going to result in a self-harm attempt or an explosion. In IFFT, we balance safety with change *very* carefully. We start with the smaller, less charged problematic behavior, improve it, get it well established as a new habit, and then work our way up the treatment hierarchy to the bigger things (e.g., not hurting themselves). It's an easy way to assess the child's readiness for change, and, just as importantly, the parents' readiness to implement change.

The pitch is made to the child by the parents in a family therapy session (with our coaching in advance) and with support from the therapist. And it's asked super nicely. Something like, "Hey, we were thinking it might be really great if you would consider showering again. What do you think about that?" I find that the vast majority of kids will agree to a request made in this way. I don't know if it's the fact that they are in session so it feels less socially acceptable to flat-out say no, or perhaps they agree to the request in session knowing full well they have no intention of actually doing it. It doesn't really matter much to me. I just want the "Okay, I'll try" because I fully intend to circle back to this quasi-commitment in subsequent sessions. And in some instances (albeit rarely) simply asking kids in session for a commitment to do something new is enough to get them to do it, or to at least give it a reasonable effort. If so, that problem is solved and then we go on to the next one up the hierarchy.

Rather than agreeing easily to the pitch, a child or teen might argue against it and say things like "You know how hard that is for me" or "I'm too tired/depressed/anxious to do that." When this occurs, we coach parents not to try to rebut the arguments and persuade because this leads to an inevitable "tug-of-war". A tug-of-war with a child is very much like the game people play on a beach—two sides line up and both pull the rope as hard as they can in hopes of bringing the opposing team over the line that runs down the middle. Every argument I've ever witnessed, both personally and professionally, involves a tug-of-war. Each person is pulling hard on the rope, throwing out argument after argument to convince the other person they're right. And what does the other person do? They pull back equally hard with their own arguments with exactly the same results. I'm certain that the parents have talked about the reasons for showering until they're blue in the face, so why bother to do it yet again? Instead, let go of the rope. The most ideal response in this situation is to matter-of-factly respond by saying, "Yeah that's true, probably not your first choice. But thanks for being open to it, and maybe just give it your best effort." If parents keep trying to talk kids into doing something they don't want to do, it just incentivizes kids to keep arguing with them in response.

But again, typically, most kids will agree to the request but then won't do it. This is not terribly surprising; remember that by this point most of the kids treated in IFFT aren't doing a whole lot of anything, and if just being nicely asked to do something worked, you wouldn't be reading this book and I'd be out of a job.

Next, in the family therapy session the following week, we ask parents to bring it up again in as friendly a way as they can: "Hey, we talked about you taking a shower every day. What happened with that?" Here the child will offer up some sort of a reason, like "I don't remember agreeing to that", "I forgot", "I tried but couldn't" and so on. We encourage parents never to argue with the reason (remember, the reason is often unreliable data). Offering to remind them to shower (or do a chore, do a little bit of homework each day, be nice, or whatever) probably won't work because it's not a forgetting problem, it's a motivation, oppositional, or anxious avoidance problem. And it treats kids like they're fragile, which I don't believe they are, including kids who are really struggling. The most ideal response to an argument as to why they didn't shower is just a simple, "Well that's okay, but how about we try this again next week?" but then to talk a bit longer about it with the therapist joining in the discussion as well.

It's what I think of as a "talk-it-to-death" strategy. It's when you bring something up to a person, over and over, nicely, to the point where they are incentivized to make the behavior change just to get you to finally shut up.

Remember, in each of these weeks there's also a lot happening behind the scenes. The child has met several times with their individual therapist, who is doing their own work on this, plus, in IFFT, kids meet weekly with a skills coach who helps them with strategies to work on their depression or anxiety, and we're assessing safety constantly.

If, after several weeks the gentle-ask strategy isn't working and the new behavior still has not occurred, we change gears and look for ways to give the child incentive to overcome or override their reluctance or avoidance. Essentially, we give them a good reason to do the thing they don't want to do, which, in many instances, entails only giving access to a device or some other preferred activity contingent on engaging in whatever behavior has been targeted for change. We'll talk more about how to do this throughout the book, but it's a highly effective strategy.

This process, repeated systematically and relentlessly over time, invariably makes it such that parents can gradually raise their expectations and parental power, allowing for an eventual return to more typical family life and a corresponding reduction in the child's mental health symptoms. It's a bit counterintuitive; behavior change results in massive changes in how a child feels (when they do better, they feel better). The stakes can be very high, however, as to some degree we are stressing a fragile system, but careful clinical attention is paid to not moving too quickly (or not quickly enough).

Language Has Power

Another part of righting the ship that can also begin at the start of treatment is helping families normalize their vocabulary on all things mental illness.

One of the unintended consequences of society's destigmatizing mental illness and psychotherapy is the amount of readily available information on various psychological disorders. Now more than ever, both parents and teenagers are much better informed about mental illness, but in ways that are not necessarily helpful. I find that many families who come into treatment have done at least some reading on childhood mental illness and its purported underlying causes. For example, most parents believe that depression is something that "happens to people" and that their child "has it." If you were to ask them why their child is depressed, most will make some kind of reference to something going biologically wrong in the brain ("a chemical imbalance").

This book is an attempt to reconceptualize much of what we know about the treatment of childhood mental illness. There are better ways to account for what is going on, which, in turn, point us in the direction of much more effective treatment.

But for now, let's just start with the use of language. The outcome of all of this Googling is that both the parents and the child have adopted much of the clinical language of my profession, and not in a good way. Yet, language has tremendous power—the words we use to describe an experience go a long way in determining how we think and feel about that experience. How parents (and therapists) speak to children, and their word choice, can have an enormous impact on how the child thinks and feels about something.

Word choice matters. A lot.

Let's take a look at some of the research in this area and figure out how we can make good use of it when it comes to treating a child's mental health condition.

Research conducted by Lindquist and Barrett at Boston College found that labeling one's unpleasant experience with emotion words can cause that emotion to occur. For example, when individuals were exposed to words relating to fear prior to listening to unpleasant music, they were more likely to subsequently engage in behaviors typically associated with fear than people who were exposed to words related to anger, or those not exposed to any emotional category labels prior to listening to the music (Lindquist & Barrett, 2008).

Elizabeth Loftus and John Palmer at the University of Washington found that language can greatly influence perceptions and memory. They hypothesized that asking leading questions would influence people's memory of an event. They asked participants to watch short clips of car accidents. One week later they asked participants to estimate the speed of motor vehicles in the accident using different forms of questions. Participants were asked how fast the cars were going when they either "smashed", "collided", "bumped", "hit", or "contacted" each other. They found that the verb choice in the question influenced the participants' perception and memory of the event. The participants in the "smashed" condition reported the highest speed estimate (40.8 mph), followed by "collided" (39.3 mph), "bumped" (38.1 mph), "hit" (34 mph), and "contacted" (31.8 mph) (Loftus & Palmer, 1974).

Martin Pickering and Simon Garrod (2004) at the University of Edinburgh found that when people are speaking to each other, one speaker often will imitate the other speaker in their volume, pitch, and tone. Speakers may also adapt similar ways of speaking in terms of grammar and word choice. I refer to this earlier in the book as "mirroring and matching." It's an unconscious tendency when speaking to someone to mirror back their emotional state and to match them in volume, pace, and intensity. Everyone does this, and once you become aware of it you'll notice this pattern all of the time. It's important for parents to be aware of this because they can use this effect to their advantage. I always recommend that parents stay "low and slow" because if they raise their voice to a kid it increases the probability of the kid raising their voice in return.

In a fascinating set of experiments, John Bargh and his colleagues at New York University conducted research on what they refer to as the "priming effect," which is the activation of unconscious concepts and stereotypes that influence behavior without the person being aware this is happening (Bargh et al., 1996). They asked the study participants to read from a larger list of neutral words that contained words typically associated with old age, such as wrinkle, old, bingo, retired, and Florida. After all the word lists had been read, study participants left the room and walked down the corridor more slowly than participants who only read lists that contained the neutral words. In another experiment, Bargh found that when participants were presented with words related to rudeness such as bold, rude, and intrude, they tended to engage in rude behaviors like interrupting the experimenter more often. When they were primed with words related to politeness, such as honor and respect, they were more polite to the experimenter.

There are also examples of how words related to mental health can influence one's perception of a negative experience. A study investigated how people perceived someone described as a "rape victim" versus a "rape survivor." Women who were described as "rape victims" were seen as more vulnerable, weak, powerless, and possessing other negative internal personal characteristics. However, when women were described as "rape survivors" they were seen as more capable and resilient. The only difference is swapping out one word for another (Hockett et al., 2014).

Ian Hacking has described what he refers to as the "classification effect," which is the tendency for people, once they are put into a classification (e.g., major depressive disorder)—especially by an authority figure such as a doctor or therapist—to behave in a manner consistent with that classification (Tsou, 2007). Hacking also states that once a "disorder" is identified and named, it can have the effect of "making up people," that is, creating a kind of person that did not exist prior to the existence of the classification (Hacking, 2006). One such example of this might be seasonal affective disorder (SAD). SAD is a pattern of major depressive disorder associated with seasonal declines in the amount of daylight. The problem is that SAD might not actually exist. A large-scale survey of over 34,000 adults used geographical location and included the actual day of the year, the latitude, and the amount of sunlight exposure, and found depression to be unrelated to any of these seasonal measures (Traffanstedt et al., 2016). The study authors conclude that "[t]he idea of seasonal depression may be strongly rooted in folk psychology, but it is not supported by objective data." Well, maybe that is the case for major depression, but what about less severe, milder feelings of depression? As it turns out, that also appears to be unrelated to season, latitude, or measures of daylight hours (LoBello & Mehta, 2019). It doesn't seem at all like a stretch to conclude that if a person has been told SAD exists and that they have it, that person has "been made," and they are highly likely to experience low mood every winter.

Over my many years in practice I have seen the word "trauma" broaden in ways that I do not believe are necessarily helpful. Many of the adolescents that I work with have adopted the word "traumatic" and expanded it to include experiences or situations that most would not consider as such in the traditional sense of the word. Many of them come into therapy and report that they've been traumatized, but when asked to describe the event itself their responses are often very surprising. One adolescent patient stated, "My gym teacher yelled at me in front of the class." While obviously not a good thing, in the past, a kid might have said that this same event made them angry or was embarrassing—words that seem much more proportional to what actually occurred.

Now I'm not in any way saying that trauma doesn't sometimes play a significant role in the development of a mental health problem; clearly, that's true. Many kids have experienced horrific events of every conceivable kind. I'm just saying the loose application of the word can have a powerful effect on how the child is going to experience an event. If experiences that are legitimately difficult or challenging are mislabeled as traumatic, this does them a disservice and can make people feel more broken, helpless, and less able to cope with negative life events. Our goal in treatment is to communicate the opposite—we want our patients to see themselves as capable. strong, and resilient, not fragile and damaged.

Now would I tell that same kid that what happened in gym class was not traumatic? Absolutely no. They'd just insist it was, and we'd be in a tug of war, which would only serve to push them deeper into their position. Instead, I would be very mindful of my word choice and most definitely not mirror back the word traumatic at any time in the conversation. I might respond with something like, "Oh no, that sounds like it was really upsetting." *Upsetting.* Or, "I bet that was super embarrassing, huh?" *Embarrassing.* I would keep using similar words throughout the conversation, still validating their experience as a challenge, but the new word choice de-energizes the event itself, thus normalizing it. I would keep my tone of voice light and easy, working hard to not match the kid if their tone was somber or overly serious. Just using a slightly lighter tone capitalizes on the mirroring effect, increasing the probability that, as the conversation unfolds, they will start to unconsciously match my tone and possibly my word choice.

I had a young adult patient who frequently used the word "depressed" to describe an experience in ways that I didn't think did him any favors. I also know that he didn't have major depressive disorder, a serious condition that can be hard to treat. He would often come into session and when I'd ask him how the previous week went, he'd say something like, "Oh Paul, my depression was really bad yesterday." The word depression gets my attention. On purpose, I'd reply by saying, "Oh no, it sounds like yesterday was a harder day than usual and you were down, yeah?" I'd keep doing this every time he'd use the word depressed (or "your mood was low") and within about 10 minutes into the session, he'd stop using the word depressed and swap it out for one of mine ("Yeah, I guess I was kinda down yesterday"). Why does this matter? Because "depressed" is a powerful word; it brings to mind unbearable sadness and misery. People associate it with something chronic and hopeless. Feeling down or having a low mood normalizes the experience—we all have down days—and it also implies that mood is just temporary and will pass. (As do all moods, both good and bad. I tell my patients that moods are like house guests—they come and visit for a while, but then eventually leave.)

This is how I advise parents when it comes to language choice. We first talk about the research on how language can change our perception, and then I encourage them to look for opportunities to de-energize and normalize their own and their child's word choice. For example, one parent told me, "She had a panic attack last night when we were talking and totally shut down." A panic attack is an actual thing (they're awful but treatable, thankfully) and I knew his daughter did not suffer from panic disorder. I suggested they consider changing their own word choice to, "She got overwhelmed when we were talking last night and then she just went quiet." It's normal for someone to get overwhelmed (a much less powerful word) and completely normal for kids to decide they just don't want to talk about something. To the daughter in that moment, it would have been helpful for the parent to say, "Alright, well I can see you're not in a space to talk right now. We can circle back to it later. I'll give you some space." No mention of panic attacks, because they were never really in the room at all.

I ask parents to just be moms and dads, and not talk like the kid's therapist. I think as a profession, we are quick to pathologize kids—to take what is often very normal teenage, human behavior, albeit sometimes exaggerated, and slap a label on it. Our word choice as therapists is equally powerful, perhaps more so because people trust that we know what we're doing.

Okay, so I've started to build an argument in favor of family-focused treatment. It's probably time for me to back up my position on this with some hard data. In the next chapter, let's take a look at what the research on family therapy tells us, and why I believe family-based treatments should be a first-line therapy for serious child and adolescent mental health problems.

Chief Takeaways from Chapter 3

For Parents

- Your child's mental health condition and accompanying symptoms are far less likely to be rooted in biology (an alleged "chemical imbalance", for example), and far more likely to be due to various situational influences affecting them currently.
- Often, parents of a child with a mental health condition begin to gradually lower their expectations of them and treat them as more fragile than they really are.
- The Principle of Least Effort tells us that people try to avoid doing hard things when they can be made easier. Kids will often cite their mental health condition as something that prevents them from meeting age-appropriate expectations.
- When parents acquiesce to this, the child's behavior is inadvertently reinforced (made stronger), providing the child with incentives not to get better (their symptoms then serve a function).
- Kids feel better when they do better, not the other way around.
- Be mindful of the power of language. Both kids and parents often begin to adopt language that magnifies a child's negative experience. For example, it is better for you to use the word "down" rather than "depressed".
- The classification effect is a phenomenon that occurs when people are put into categories and then act in ways consistent with the classification (a diagnosis, for example).

For Clinicians

- Situational influences deserve significant clinical attention because they are very likely at the root of the child or teen's current mental health struggles.
- Encourage parents to have high expectations of their child, and to be mindful of acquiescing and thus reinforcing the very behaviors they are trying to change.
- Start with the "low hanging fruit" and consider using the Gentle Ask strategy.
- Many of the symptoms and behaviors exhibited by a child or teen serve a function that, once identified, can be disrupted.
- Patients are not going to feel better until they do better. You have to target behavior change as a priority, because if you just wait for them to feel better in the hopes that their behavior will improve, you're going to be waiting a long time.
- Be mindful of your own participation in the classification effect. I think it's time that, as a profession, we stop "making people." In my opinion, we as therapists place far more stock in a child or teen's diagnosis than we should.

References

Bargh, J. A., Chen, M., & Burrows, L. (1996). Automaticity of social behavior: Direct effects of trait construct and stereotype activation on action. *Journal of Personality and Social Psychology*, 71(2), 230–244. 10.1037/0022-3514.71.2.230

Cialdini, R. (2009). *Influence: Science and practice* (5th ed.). Allyn and Bacon.

Hacking, I. (2006, August 17). Making up people. *London Review of Books*, 28(16). https://www.lrb.co.uk/the-paper/v28/n16/ian-hacking/making-up-people

Hagura, N., Haggard, P., & Diedrichsen, J. (2017). Perceptual decisions are biased by the cost to act. *eLife*, 6, Article e18422. 10.7554/eLife.18422

Hockett, J. M., McGraw, L. K., & Saucier, D. A. (2014). A "rape victim" by any other name: The effects of labels on individuals' rate-related perceptions. In H. Pishwa & R. Schulze (Eds.), *The expression of inequality in interaction: Power, dominance, and status* (pp. 81–104). John Benjamins Publishing Company.

Lindquist, K. A., & Barrett, L. F. (2008). Constructing emotion: The experience of fear as a conceptual act. *Psychological Science*, 19(9), 898–903. 10.1111/j.1467-9280.2008.02174.x

LoBello, S. G., & Mehta, S. (2019). No evidence of seasonal variation in mild forms of depression. *Journal of Behavior Therapy and Experimental Psychiatry*, 62, 72–79. 10.1016/j.jbtep.2018.09.003

Loftus, E. F., & Palmer, J. C. (1974). Reconstruction of automobile destruction: An example of the interaction between language and memory. *Journal of Verbal Learning & Verbal Behavior*, 13(5), 585–589. 10.1016/S0022-5371 (74)80011-3

Pickering, M. J., & Garrod, S. (2004). Toward a mechanistic psychology of dialogue. *Behavioral and Brain Sciences*, 27(2), 169–190. 10.1017/S0140525X04 000056

Traffanstedt, M. K., Mehta, S., & LoBello, S. G. (2016). Major depression with seasonal variation: Is it a valid construct? *Clinical Psychological Science*, 4(5), 825–834. 10.1177/2167702615615867

Tsou, J. Y. (2007). Hacking on the looping effects of psychiatric classifications: What is an interactive and indifferent kind? *International Studies in the Philosophy of Science*, 21(3), 329–344. 10.1080/02698590701589601

4 The Case for Family-Focused Treatment

I am obviously a great proponent of family therapy and family-based treatments. I should probably begin by differentiating the two terms, as I don't see them as being exactly the same thing.

I think of family therapy in the more transitional sense, as you likely do as well. Simply put, when I use the term family therapy, I am referring to a session in which the family and the child are together in the same room. These sessions tend to focus on helping families improve their communication, troubleshoot and resolve either historical or day-to-day conflicts, negotiate and reach agreements on various family issues, and so on. It's basically getting everyone in the same room, talking and trying to work things out without anyone coming to blows.

The term family-based treatment is broader and often includes quite a bit more than just family therapy sessions. Parents often seek out treatment because their child or teen has developed not just a mental health condition but a set of behaviors that go along with that condition and that are almost always very distressing. Much of the focus of treatment, therefore, is on these behaviors with the goal of ameliorating them over time. Any form of treatment that does not positively change behavior in a significant way is going to be a very unsatisfying treatment indeed.

So to avoid confusion, from here on in this book I'll use the term family-focused treatment, which encompasses both family therapy and family-based treatment interventions.

So how do you change a child's problematic behavior? I strongly believe that the most efficient and effective way to change another person's behavior, whether it's a child or another adult, is by first changing one's own behavior. In Chapter 2, we learned a great deal about the power of social influences. I'm going to show parents and clinicians how to harness its power to help a child during the period of their lives in which they clearly need it the most.

I also believe that the single most important factor determining how a child will behave again after a problem behavior has occurred is how a

DOI: 10.4324/9781003397366-6

parent or other adult responds to that behavior. To put it simply, parents are massively powerful change agents. But parents generally don't see it that way, or at least not at the beginning of treatment. In fact, it's the reverse—parents often feel completely powerless, and understandably so, since virtually everything they have tried clearly has not worked.

I believe an important part of family-focused treatment is putting an emphasis on changing parents' behavior in ways that are highly beneficial to the child or teen. This would include weekly parent sessions (in addition to family therapy sessions) where the content is geared toward letting go of habits or responses that clearly aren't working and replacing those with a new set of skills, strategies, and interventions that work much better. The parents' therapist has an interesting and challenging job—we are tasked with changing a child or adolescent's behavior indirectly by changing the parents' behavior. Not an easy trick, but in most cases, it is highly effective.

There is no one who will ever love a child as much or in the same way as they are loved by their own parents. *No one.* As such, in my view, parents are the single most powerful change agents in a child's life. (Well, except for negative peers but more on that later.) Not that therapists aren't change agents; we are, but our ability to change a child's behavior pales in comparison with a child's own parents. We just don't have that same kind of power. Consequently, as a therapist, I will capitalize on the power of parents to influence their child's behavior to my (and their) full advantage.

So, here's the thing. I am about to share with you what I believe is the best-kept secret both within and outside the mental health community: There are approximately 40 years of accumulated research clearly demonstrating that family-focused treatments are effective for children and adolescents with moderate to severe mental health conditions. Study after study has been published in highly reputable, scientific journals.

I'm willing to bet if you are a parent reading this book you probably weren't aware of this. I'd also be willing to bet that most therapists reading this book also likely didn't know that. (Unless you're a family therapy nerd like me, but I don't think there are a lot of us in the universe.)

And here's another interesting piece of information that health insurance companies have not fully dialed into yet: Not only are family therapy and family-focused treatments supported by research, but they are also cost-effective.

D. Russell Crane and his colleague Jacob Christenson (2012) summarized the results of 22 studies concluding that family treatment results in a reduction in healthcare costs. For example, Crane and his colleagues (2005) used the state of Kansas Medicaid data to examine costs for treating children and adolescents with conduct disorder (kids who engage in extreme, often hostile, delinquent-type behavior). A total of 3,763 adolescents received either in-office family therapy (N = 164), in-office individual therapy (N = 3,096), or in-home family therapy (N = 503). Their results indicate that, compared with healthcare costs for those receiving just individual therapy, costs for children who received family therapy were 32% lower. For those who received in-home family therapy, the costs were even better: 85% lower. Note that despite the established efficacy of family-focused treatments, the vast majority of children in the sample (82.2%) were still provided with just individual therapy.

Where Our Mental Healthcare System Gets It Wrong

There exists a peculiar and long-standing bias in our healthcare system, at least our current system in the U.S., that when a child or teen struggles with a mental health condition such as depression, self-harm, anxiety, and so on, no one thinks about family-focused treatment as a first-line intervention. That is despite four decades of research demonstrating that it works and that it's cost-effective. Instead, we treat kids as if their problems and issues exist somewhere inside of them—something broken that needs fixing. Services are delivered to them individually. They are sent to weekly individual therapy, prescribed psychiatric medication, put in psychiatric hospitals or partial hospitals (day programs), or even sent to residential treatment, the most individually focused treatment of all.

Children and adolescents do not live their lives in a vacuum. Their thoughts, emotions, hopes, dreams, and fears all exist within the contexts or situations in which they find themselves. These situational variables exert a massive influence on our kids and their well-being. I believe there is nothing wrong with the child per se, but there can be many things wrong with the various relevant situations and influences that can make for a very unhappy child. I tell families all the time that this isn't a kid problem to solve; *it's a family problem to solve.* We'll talk much more about changing situational influences in the next chapter and throughout the rest of this book.

And I'm not saying that we shouldn't send children to individual therapy. Of course, we should, especially in the early stages of a developing mental health problem. Many children and teens need only individual therapy and benefit quite nicely from it. But in the more serious cases, kids who don't respond to therapy and are getting worse, individual therapy alone or more services directed individually at the child seem, to me, no longer appropriate.

Rather than a first-line treatment, the inclusion of family-focused treatment is often an afterthought or a last-ditch effort despite its documented efficacy. That's the first part of the problem. The second part of the problem is that there are far more individual therapists than there are family therapists. Most therapists just don't do family therapy. My own experience is that individual therapy is a lot easier. You have only one personality in the room to deal with, not several. There's nothing more enjoyable than spending an hour with an 11-year-old, they're super fun (well, an hour with a five-year-old is, in my opinion, even better). A family therapy session is hard; it's like a fast-moving volcanic river that can engulf the therapist at any moment. Many families run extremely hot, and it takes a very skilled therapist and a lot of hard work to keep things from going haywire.

In this chapter, I'm going to "show you the money" on the importance of family-focused treatment. I tend to be somewhat skeptical by nature and I often need a lot of convincing, so perhaps you do too. I'm going to begin by walking you through some of my own research and what I've learned about the relationship between how well families function and children's mental health. After we lay that groundwork, I'll walk you through the best-known, most-researched, family-focused models of treatment currently available and highlight each model's most important research findings.

My Research on Family Functioning

Just a quick disclaimer here before we get started.

I consider myself to be a family therapist first and a researcher as a very distant second. Before starting work on my doctorate, I had already been working in mental health and with children for quite a while. Graduate school requires reading a lot of research, and I developed a keen appreciation for it. My dissertation was such that I was able to gather quite a bit of interesting data on kids and their families which I was able to publish as a paper (Sunseri, 2001).

I was heavily involved in the residential care industry at this time in my career. I had worked in many different types of programs and eventually founded and oversaw two residential treatment programs for children and adolescents with very serious mental health conditions. Back then, in the 1980s and 1990s, the residential community didn't really involve families much in their children's treatment or do much family therapy. (Quite shockingly, to this day, many still don't do family therapy, or they pay what seems to me only token attention to it.) I think most of us working in the field knew that families played an important role in what was going on with the child, but none of us, including me, were quite sure how important family therapy was or even knew how to do it halfway decently. As it turns out, a lot of kids back then did not get better in residential treatment, so there you go.

I was on the hunt for another research project, and I wanted to know more about the role families (parents) play in their children's mental health conditions, especially children needing residential treatment. As luck would have it, I was granted access to a large data set on children and teens treated in a large number of residential programs over a six-year period, compiled by an industry association. Miraculously, the association let me study the data it had collected, which was surprising because it showed that most of these kids at that time didn't get any better. The association figured that out well before I did, ultimately resulting in its pulling the plug on data collection.

How large was the sample? Big. A little more than 8,900 kids in treatment. The association had created this very cool, very comprehensive survey that was filled out on each kid at the time they entered the program and again at the time they were discharged. It asked all sorts of interesting things, such as scores that rated the severity of the child's behavior problems from admission to discharge, and scores on something called the Global Assessment of Functioning Scale (Aas, 2010), which measures the child's overall functioning. The survey also showed which kids graduated from the program successfully versus those who left because they weren't getting any better.

But, best of all is that the survey included a measure of how well each kid's family functioned along various dimensions: the ability to solve family-related problems, how well they managed stress and conflict, the parents' general parenting skills, and more. Each of these areas was given a numerical score, so, ultimately, I was able to classify families into three distinct groups: high-functioning, intermediate-functioning, and low-functioning.

Guess what I found? On every single measure I looked at, kids from low-functioning families (poor communication, lots of conflict, and little collaboration) were the worst off. They had the most serious behavior problems relative to kids with intermediate- or high-functioning families, both at the start of treatment and still at the time of discharge, and many of them got demonstrably worse over the course of treatment. The vast majority of kids with low-functioning families also did not graduate from treatment and instead were asked to leave due to challenging behavior. This pattern, that is, kids with low-functioning families doing badly, those from intermediate-functioning families doing somewhat better, and those from high-functioning families doing the best, held up over and over with every single analysis I performed (Sunseri, 2004).

Here are two examples. Figure 4.1 shows mean (average) scores on a measure of depression and Figure 4.2 shows scores on suicidal thoughts (the higher the bar, the more serious the problem). Notice that scores are highest for children and teens with the lowest-functioning families, but the scores get progressively better as family functioning gets better.

All of this was stunning to me. Even though those of us who worked with children with serious mental health problems intuitively knew that how well families got along and interacted was important, I actually had no idea it would turn out to be this important.

SEVERITY OF DEPRESSION AND HOW WELL THE FAMILY FUNCTIONS

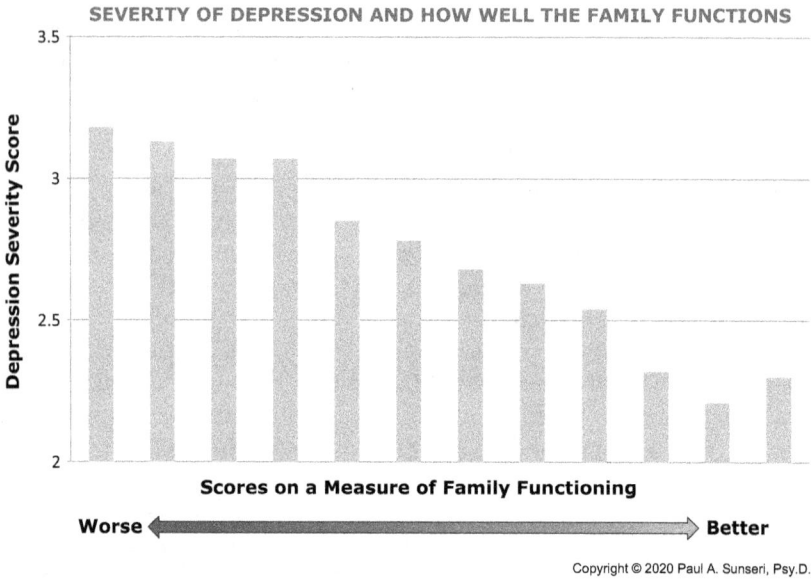

Copyright © 2020 Paul A. Sunseri, Psy.D.

Figure 4.1 The relationship between family functioning and the severity of depression in children.

SEVERITY OF SUICIDAL THOUGHTS AND HOW WELL THE FAMILY FUNCTIONS

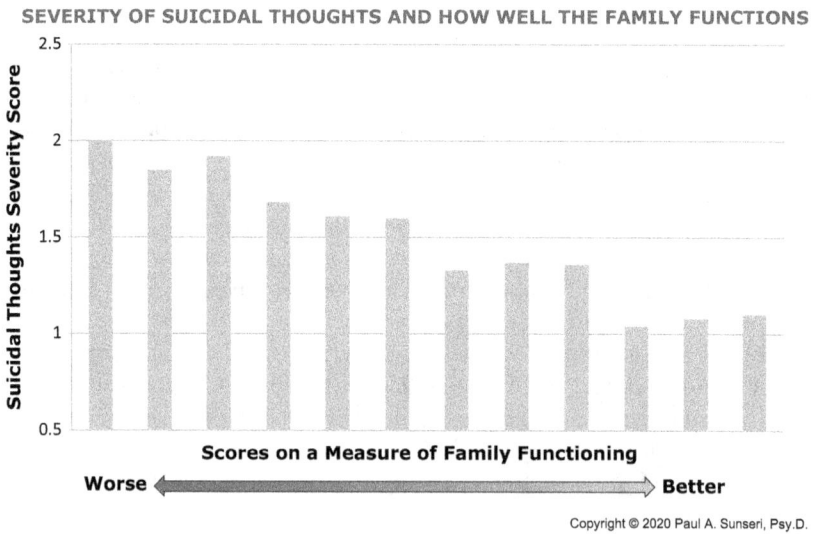

Copyright © 2020 Paul A. Sunseri, Psy.D.

Figure 4.2 The relationship between family functioning and the severity of suicidal thoughts in children.

But wait, maybe I got this all wrong somehow. Maybe I made a mistake, or mistakes, in my analyses, or perhaps there was something unique to this data set, or the way the data was collected that made it look like something it wasn't. I have since presented these findings at many conferences and I keep expecting someone in the audience to someday raise their hand and tell me that I got it all wrong and explain to me why. But nobody ever has.

This kept nagging at me for years. I finally decided to do something about it, so I set out to prove my own research wrong.

I approached another association of programs, this time in another state, that had been collecting its own data on a large number of kids treated in various residential programs in that area. How large? This time just a shade over 18,000 kids. And for those of you who don't really follow research, that's considered a very large sample. So: different kids, different time period, different state, and different programs. To make this all the more exciting (to me anyway), this association used a completely different way to measure family functioning, but one that still allowed me to group every kid's family into the same three categories: low-functioning, intermediate-functioning, and high-functioning (Sunseri, 2020).

So I crunched all of the data, and as you've probably already figured out, I found *exactly the same thing*. Children and adolescents with low-functioning families struggled the most, those with intermediate-functioning families less so, and those with high-functioning families the least.

So that you don't think I'm the only one saying this, other research points us in a similar direction. In a review of 98 studies of predictors and moderators of childhood anxiety, baseline family functioning also consistently predicted youth mental health outcomes (Compton et al., 2014). Additionally, improvements in family functioning that occur over the course of treatment have direct clinical relevance. Laura Mills and her colleagues (Mills et al., 2022) report that the strength of the relationship between improved family functioning and positive changes in a child's mental health condition are profound: a 25-point improvement on a standardized measure of behavior was found for every one unit of improvement in family functioning.

Now what to do with all of this and how can we use what I, and others, have learned in a way that helps children and families?

First, although there is a clear and very robust association between how well families function and the severity of a child's mental health condition and the behavioral difficulties that accompany that condition, I can't tell you what direction that goes in. It's the correlation-is-not-causation argument you've probably heard of (just because two things go together you can't say that one necessarily causes the other). So, I don't know if families that struggle with their ability to communicate, navigate conflict well, negotiate, and solve problems collaboratively are causing kids to struggle more, or if having kids with very challenging behavior results in more family conflict, poorer communication, and so on.

Both explanations seem entirely plausible to me. And, while I don't have the evidence to know for sure, common sense tells me that both dynamics are likely coming into play to varying degrees with every family that has a child with a mental health condition. Difficult-to-parent kids with serious behavior problems can cause an awful lot of conflict in a family, and a worsening of communication, and very bad communication can cause an awful lot of conflict and upset in the kid.

From a clinical perspective, here's what I think makes the most sense: therapists should work hard on improving both simultaneously. Good family treatment should have as its aim the improvement of family functioning. The child can only stand to benefit from teaching families how to communicate better; be mindful of how to approach a problem or an issue in a way that doesn't lead to unnecessary conflict or an escalation; and work to improve problem-solving, negotiation, and collaboration skills. Similarly, a family's functioning can only stand to benefit by implementing targeted and effective strategies to reduce the severity of the child's behavioral issues.

Evidence-Based Models of Family-Focused Treatments

I mentioned previously that about 40 years of research documents the efficacy of family-focused treatments. In the remainder of this chapter, I'm going to walk you through seven existing family treatment models and summarize the relevant research that has been conducted on each. The treatment models that follow have substantial empirical support, plus each includes a quality-control element: therapists who implement the model in real-world conditions are properly trained, supervised, and ultimately certified in its delivery before being unleashed on the world.

Functional Family Therapy

Functional family therapy (FFT), developed in the late 1960s by James Alexander, is a model of treatment developed for children and adolescents with disruptive behavior problems (Sexton & Turner, 2010). Michael Robbins and colleagues (2016) describe FFT as providing a framework for understanding family relationship patterns and identifying the meaning and function of behaviors within the family. Treatment interventions are designed to increase adaptive behaviors and decrease or eliminate maladaptive behaviors within the family context. FFT is a manualized family-based intervention program (which means that there is a prescriptive, step-by-step process in its delivery). FFT is a short-term intervention based on family systems theory and consisting of approximately 30 hours of treatment. FFT is designed to address family dysfunction by recognizing and changing maladaptive family communication patterns, training family members to negotiate effectively, set clear boundaries regarding rules and responsibilities, and expand changes to community contexts and other relationships (Weisman & Montgomery, 2019). Therapists delivering FFT use directive teaching, as well as creating, leading, modeling, and reviewing in-session tasks. Therapists also assign and review homework with clients (California Evidence-Based Clearing House for Child Welfare, 2019).

Numerous studies have shown FFT to be effective (Becker & Oxman, 2008; ,Weisman & Montgomery, 2019). Thomas Sexton from Indiana University and Charles Turner from the Oregon Research Institute (Sexton & Turner, 2011) compared FFT with probation services for at-risk youth. FFT was effective in reducing behavioral problems, but, unsurprisingly, only when therapists adhered to the FFT model (what's known as "treatment fidelity"). FFT demonstrated statistically significant reductions in subsequent felonies (35%), violent crime (30%), and a smaller, more modest reduction in misdemeanor crimes (21%), compared with treatment as usual. In another study, Dan Hartnett and his colleagues at University College Dublin (2017) conducted a systematic review of published and unpublished articles of 14 studies containing 18 comparisons between FFT and other forms of treatment including CBT, other forms of family therapy, and individual and group therapy for adolescents demonstrating disruptive behavior and substance use disorders. FFT was more effective than these well-defined alternative treatments. Robbins and colleagues (2016) reviewed four decades' worth of research studies on FFT, demonstrating strong efficacy with delinquent and substance-using youth, including serious habitual offenders.

Multidimensional Family Therapy

Multidimensional family therapy (MDFT), was developed by Howard Liddle, professor of public health sciences, psychology, and counseling psychology at the University of Miami Miller School of Medicine. MDFT is a research-driven intervention for adolescent substance abuse and associated mental health and behavioral problems. MDFT uses a "contextual conceptual framework" (understanding something within its context). MDFT assesses and intervenes in four areas: (1) the adolescent as an individual and a member of a family and peer network; (2) the parents, both as individual adults and their role as caregivers; (3) the family environment and family relationships, as manifested by daily family interactions patterns; and (4) extrafamilial sources of influence such as peers, school and juvenile justice. MDFT establishes individual relationships with the parent and teen, works with each individually in sessions, targets family interactional changes, and also works with individuals and parents via the teen and family's social context. MDFT not only works with the parents individually but also focuses on working with the teen alone, apart from the parent sessions, and apart from the family sessions (Liddle, 2010).

MDFT is one of the most well-researched therapies for adolescent substance abuse and delinquency (Liddle, 2010). MDFT has shown outcomes superior to several other well-established treatments (see Liddle, 2010 for a review of these studies). Ten completed randomized controlled trials have tested MDFT against a variety of therapies for adolescents with drug problems. MDFT has demonstrated superior outcomes to several other well-established treatments, including a psychoeducational multi-family group intervention, peer-group treatment, individual CBT, and residential treatment.

Multisystemic Family Therapy

Multisystemic therapy (MST) was developed by Scott Henggeler in the 1970s. MST is an evidence-based treatment for youth and their families with challenging clinical problems, and it uses a social and ecological framework. MST asserts that parents and caregivers are the key to achieving and sustaining positive long-term results, and its interventions focus intensely on empowering parents. MST targets risk factors within the family, peer group, school, and neighborhood. The aim is to create a context that supports adaptive, rather than maladaptive, child and parent behavior (Henggeler & Schaeffer, 2016). MST is based on the theory that adolescent delinquency is associated with an accumulation of risk factors for criminal behavior, which includes individual, family, peer, school, and neighborhood characteristics. MST asserts that these factors must be targeted simultaneously because human behavior develops in multiple contexts (situations). MST mainly focuses on improving family functioning, and it theorizes that improvements in family functioning lead to improvements in peer relationships, school functioning, and participation in the community (Van der Stouwe et al., 2014).

MST has a large body of evidence to support its efficacy. Rigorous efficacy trials clearly showed MST has achieved favorable outcomes with youth with very serious clinical problems and with their families, including chronic criminality and violence (see Henggeler, 2012 for a review of these studies). Several studies, including 25 published random controlled trials

(RCTs), support the effectiveness of MST in treating very challenging clinical problems including violence, substance abuse, and serious emotional disturbance (Henggeler & Schaeffer, 2016). The first meta-analysis on MST (a type of study that combines the results of multiple other studies) was conducted by Nicola Curtis and her colleagues in 2004 (Curtis et al., 2004). It was found that MST was more effective than the treatment-as-usual group. MST had the most effect on family relationships compared with individual adjustment and peer relationships.

Brief Strategic Family Therapy

Brief strategic family therapy (BSFT) was developed within the Hispanic and Latino communities by José Szapocznik, chair emeritus professor and director of the Center for Family Studies at the University of Miami. BSFT focuses on developing an understanding of the nature of maladaptive family interactions and their relationship to the family system, using purposeful and problem-focused interventions. The focus is on social interaction among family members (Szapocznik & Williams, 2000). BSFT targets family interaction patterns that are the most directly relevant to behavior issues targeted for change. A maladaptive family structure is seen as an important contributor to the occurrence and maintenance of behavior problems, drug abuse, and other antisocial behavior. The therapist alters family interactions so that the parent becomes the source of support. Positive changes are created in family patterns of interactions, thereby improving family functioning.

Szapocznik and his colleagues (1989) compared BSFT with psychodynamic child therapy and a nontreatment control condition. The sample consisted of 69 Hispanic and Latino boys aged six to 12 with behavioral and emotional problems. Results demonstrated that BSFT and psychodynamic child therapy were equally effective at reducing behavioral and emotional problems and improving functioning. However, BSFT brought about significant improvement in family functioning at the one-year follow-up, whereas the psychodynamic condition and control condition did not. This study demonstrated that BSFT is a promising family-focused approach to treating Hispanic youth with behavior problems and drug abuse. In another study, Daniel Santisteban and colleagues examined the efficacy of BSFT in reducing behavior problems. BSFT was compared with a control condition delivered in a group format (Santisteban et al., 2003). They found adolescents in the BSFT condition showed significant reductions in conduct disorder and aggression from pre- to post-treatment.

The reader will notice that most of the outcome studies on the preceding models involved youth in the juvenile justice system. These are generally adolescents who exhibit conduct problems (impulsive, high-risk, rule-breaking behavior) along with substance use. If you are a parent reading this and your child doesn't exactly fit this clinical picture, rest easy. This population of adolescents is notoriously difficult to treat, as you might imagine. I have great respect for the aforementioned model developers, as they chose to work with a group of kids from whom most would shy away. And it seems very reasonable to me that if these family-focused models could achieve such great outcomes with this very difficult-to-treat population, I feel confident they would also work very well for everyone else.

Attachment-Based Family Therapy

Attachment-based family therapy (ABFT), was developed by Guy Diamond, Suzanne Levy, and Gary Diamond. ABFT is a treatment grounded in attachment theory and using an interpersonal trauma-focused approach in treating depression, suicidality, and trauma among adolescents. ABFT focuses on interpersonal risk factors for depression. The goal of ABFT is that parents become someone the adolescent can turn to for support, comfort, and guidance (Diamond et al., 2003). Attachment theory asserts that human beings innately strive for connection with others. When a parent appropriately responds to their children's attachment needs, children generally develop a secure attachment (Bowlby, 1969, 1988, as cited in Diamond et al., 2003). The first half of ABFT treatment focuses on helping the adolescent identify and discuss past and present family conflicts or events that have ruptured the attachment bond and damaged trust between family members. The therapist helps parents tolerate and acknowledge these ruptures and assists them in apologizing for their contribution to these attachment failures. The second half of treatment focuses on promoting adolescent autonomy, for example, improving school performance, finding employment, and getting involved in school activities (Diamond et al., 2003).

ABFT has been found to be a promising treatment when used with depressed adolescents (Diamond et al., 2003). Empirical support was found in various other studies as well (see Diamond et al., 2016 for a review of these studies). Diamond and his colleagues (2010) conducted a study to measure the effectiveness of ABFT compared with enhanced usual care (EUC—a variation on treatment as usual). The study concluded that youth treated with ABFT had significantly greater and faster reductions in suicidal ideation during treatment compared with EUC. These differences persisted at follow-up, which occurred at six weeks, 12 weeks, and 24 weeks.

Emotionally Focused Family Therapy and Emotion-Focused Family Therapy

I'm going to put these last two together, not just because they have very similar names, but because they do not yet have the same degree of empirical support as the other models of family-focused treatment. Both have published research; not as much, but I suspect more research will be forthcoming.

Emotionally Focused Family Therapy (EFFT), developed by Sue Johnson, conceptualizes children's behaviors in terms of attachment needs of comfort and support (Wittenborn et al., 2006). Emotionally focused therapists understand distress in terms of attachment dilemmas or ineffective responses to attachment needs. Johnson is also the developer of EFT for couples, which does have substantial empirical support (Johnson et al., 1999).

Emotion-Focused Family Therapy, developed by Adele Lafrance, allows parents to take significant roles in their children's recovery. *This* EFFT focuses on building connection among family members and fostering resiliency. Research has found that parents of children with severe eating disorders or other mental health problems experienced a significant increase in parental self-efficacy and more positive beliefs regarding their role in their children's recovery after a two-day intervention with Emotion-Focused Family Therapy (Robinson et al., 2016; Strahan et al., 2017).

Accessing These Models for Your Own Family

These evidence-based models of family-focused treatment can be accessed right now by families in distress. A quick Google search of each should lead you to certified organizations and providers, so, hopefully, one can be found near you. I do not know what each of their policies is, relative to telehealth, but perhaps this is an option if in-person treatment is not. If this doesn't work, many therapists who began their careers in nonprofit community mental health organizations have been trained in at least one of the models, so perhaps you can locate one who is now in private practice.

If you are a therapist, and if you have not done so already, I highly recommend that you try to become certified in one of these models. Family therapy is very challenging, as you know, and it's always helpful to have a clinical roadmap to follow. If you're not able to become certified for whatever reason, each of these models has a textbook that outlines its treatment approach in much more detail than I have provided here.

In the next chapter, we'll be doing a deep dive into the model I have developed: intensive family-focused therapy (IFFT). IFFT has some similarities to the models described in this chapter, but is quite different in other ways that I think you'll find quite interesting.

Chief Takeaways from Chapter 4

For Parents

- In a family-focused approach, you are the key to positively influencing your child, and a good therapist will help you harness that power to its fullest extent.
- Family-focused treatment is the best-kept secret in the world: 40 years of research shows it works.
- Child or teen mental illness isn't a kid problem to solve; *it's a family problem to solve.*
- If your family learns how to better communicate and solve problems together, your child's behavioral issues will likely improve.
- There are many, very good evidence-based family therapy models that you can access right now.

For Clinicians

- The best way to change a child for the better is by changing the ways in which their family responds to them.
- If a child isn't benefitting from individual therapy, strongly consider adding a family component rather than adding other individually directed services.
- Help spread the word: Let's make family-focused therapy a first-line treatment.
- When family functioning improves, the child's behavior also improves; the reverse is likely true as well.
- Consider getting certified in one of the many existing family therapy models, or at the very least, become very well acquainted with one.

Bonus Tip for Insurance Companies

- Research shows that family-focused therapy reduces healthcare costs and that it's highly effective.

References

Aas, I. H. M. (2010). Global assessment of functioning (GAF): Properties and frontier of current knowledge. *Annals of General Psychiatry*, 9, Article 20. 10.1186/1744-859X-9-20

Becker, L. A., & Oxman, A. D. (2008). Overviews of reviews. In J. P. T. Higgins & S. Green (Eds.), *Cochrane handbook for systematic reviews of interventions: Cochrane book series*. Wiley-Blackwell.

Compton, S. N., Peris, T. S., Almirall, D., Birmaher, B., Sherrill, J., Kendall, P. C., March, J. S., Gosch, E. A., Ginsburg, G. S., Rynn, M. A., Piacentini, J. C., McCracken, J. T., Keeton, C. P., Suveg, C. M., Aschenbrand, S. G., Sakolsky, D., Iyengar, S., Walkup, J. T., & Albano, A. M. (2014). Predictors and moderators of treatment response in childhood anxiety disorders: Results from the CAMS trial. *Journal of Consulting and Clinical Psychology*, 82(2), 212–224. 10.1037/a0035458

Crane, D. R., & Christenson, J. D. (2012). A summary report of the cost-effectiveness of the profession and practice of marriage and family therapy. *Contemporary Family Therapy: An International Journal*, 34(2), 204–216. 10.1007/s10591-012-9187-5

Crane, D. R., Hillin, H. H., & Jakubowski, S. F. (2005). Costs of treating conduct disordered Medicaid youth with and without family therapy. *The American Journal of Family Therapy*, 33(5), 403–413. 10.1080/01926180500276810

Curtis, N. M., Ronan, K. R., & Borduin, C. M. (2004). Multisystemic treatment: A meta-analysis of outcome studies. *Journal of Family Psychology*, 18(3), 411–419. 10.1037/0893-3200.18.3.411

Diamond, G. S., Wintersteen, M. B., Brown, G. K., Diamond, G. M., Gallop, R., Shelef, K., & Levy, S. (2010). Attachment-based family therapy for adolescents with suicidal ideation: A randomized controlled trial. *Journal of the American Academy of Child and Adolescent Psychiatry*, 9(2), 122–131. 10.1097/00004583-201002000-00006

Diamond, G., Russon, J., & Levy, S. (2016). Attachment-based family therapy: A review of the empirical support. *Family Process*, 55(3), 595–610. 10.1111/famp.12241

Diamond, G., Siqueland, L., & Diamond, G. M. (2003). Attachment-based family therapy for depressed adolescents: Programmatic treatment development. *Clinical Child and Family Psychology Review*, 6(2), 107–127. 10.1023/a:1023782510786

Hartnett, D., Carr, A., Hamilton, E., & O'Reilly, G. (2017). The effectiveness of functional family therapy for adolescent behavioral and substance misuse problems: A meta-analysis. *Family Process*, 56(3), 607–619. 10.1111/famp.12256

Henggeler, S. W. (2012). Multisystemic therapy: Clinical foundations and research outcomes. *Psychosocial Intervention*, 21(2), 181–193. 10.5093/in2012a12

Henggeler, S. W., & Schaeffer, C. M. (2016). Multisystemic therapy: Clinical overview, outcomes, and implementation research. *Family Process*, 55(3), 514–528. 10.1111/famp.12232

Johnson, S. M., Hunsley, J., Greenberg, L., & Schindler, D. (1999). Emotionally focused couples therapy: Status and challenges. *Clinical Psychology: Science and Practice, 6*(1), 67–79. 10.1093/clipsy.6.1.67

Liddle, H. A. (2010). Multidimensional family therapy: A science-based treatment system. *Australian and New Zealand Journal of Family Therapy, 31*(2), 133–148. 10.1375/anft.31.2.133

Mills, L., Hall, J., Ridenour, A., & Murphy, M. (2022). The importance of parent engagement in outdoor behavioural health programs for youth. *Journal of Therapeutic Schools and Programs, 14*(1), 150–169.

Robbins, M. S., Alexander, J. F., Turner, C. W., & Hollimon, A. (2016). Evolution of functional family therapy as an evidence-based practice for adolescents with disruptive behavior problems. *Family Process, 55*(3), 543–557. 10.1111/famp.12230

Robinson, A. L., Dolhanty, J., Stillar, A., Henderson, K., & Mayman, S. (2016). Emotion-focused family therapy for eating disorders across the lifespan: A pilot study of a 2-day transdiagnostic intervention for parents. *Clinical Psychology & Psychotherapy, 23*(1), 10.1002/cpp.1933

Santisteban, D. A., Coatsworth, J. D., Perez-Vidal, A., Kurtines, W. M., Schwartz, S. J., LaPerriere, A., & Szapocznik, J. (2003). Efficacy of brief strategic family therapy in modifying Hispanic adolescent behavior problems and substance use. *Journal of Family Psychology, 17*(1), 121–133. 10.1037/0893-3200.17.1.121

Sexton, T., & Turner, C. W. (2010). The effectiveness of functional family therapy for youth with behavioral problems in a community practice setting. *Journal of Family Psychology, 24*(3), 339–348. 10.1037/a0019406

Sexton, T., & Turner, C. W. (2011). The effectiveness of functional family therapy for youth with behavioral problems in a community practice setting. *Couple and Family Psychology: Research and Practice, 1*(S), 3–15. https://doi.org/10.1037/2160-4096.1.S.3

Strahan, E. J., Stillar, A., Files, N., Nash, P., Scarborough, J., Connors, L., Gusella, J., Henderson, K., Mayman, S., Marchand, P., Orr, E. S., Dolhanty, A., & Lafrance, A. (2017). Increasing parental self-efficacy with emotion-focused family therapy for eating disorders: A process model. *Person-Centered & Experiential Psychotherapies, 16*(3), 256–269. 10.1080/14779757.2017.1330703

Sunseri, P. A. (2001). The prediction of unplanned discharge from residential treatment. *Child & Youth Care Forum, 30*(5), 283–303. 10.1023/A:1014477327436

Sunseri, P. A. (2004). Family functioning and residential treatment outcomes. *Residential Treatment for Children & Youth, 22*(1), 33–53. 10.1300/J007v22n01_03

Sunseri, P. A. (2020). Hidden figures: Is improving family functioning a key to better treatment outcomes for seriously mentally ill children? *Residential Treatment for Children & Youth, 37*(1), 46–64. 10.1080/0886571X.2019.1589405

Szapocznik, J., & Williams, R. A. (2000). Brief strategic family therapy: Twenty-five years of interplay among theory, research and practice in adolescent behavior problems and drug abuse. *Clinical Child and Family Psychology Review, 3*(2), 117–134. 10.1023/a:1009512719808

Szapocznik, J., Rio, A., Murray, E., Cohen, R., Scopetta, M., Rivas-Vazquez, A., Hervis, O., Posada, V., & Kurtines, W. (1989). Structural family versus psychodynamic child therapy for problematic Hispanic boys. *Journal of Consulting and Clinical Psychology, 57*(5), 571–578. 10.1037/0022-006X.57.5.571

The California Evidence-Based Clearinghouse for Child Welfare. (2019, July). *Functional family therapy child welfare.* Retrieved November 10, 2022, from https://www.cebc4cw.org/program/functional-family-therapy-child-welfare/

Van der Stouwe, T., Asscher, J. J., Stams, G. J. J. M., Deković, M., & van der Laan, P. H. (2014). The effectiveness of multisystemic therapy (MST): A meta-analysis. *Clinical Psychology Review, 34*(6), 468–481. 10.1016/j.cpr.2014.06.006

Weisman, C. B., & Montgomery, P. (2019). Functional family therapy (FFT) for behavior disordered youth aged 10–18: An overview of reviews. *Research on Social Work Practice, 29*(3), 333–346. 10.1177/1049731518792309

Wittenborn, A. K., Faber, A. J., Harvey, A. M., & Thomas, V. K. (2006). Emotionally focused family therapy and play therapy techniques. *The American Journal of Family Therapy, 34*(4), 333–342. 10.1080/01926180600553472

5 Intensive Family-Focused Therapy (IFFT)

This chapter will provide the reader with an overview of the theoretical lens and the structure of intensive family-focused therapy (IFFT), a model of family treatment that I have developed for children and adolescents with serious mental health conditions.

I refer to the model as "transdiagnostic," which means that the children and adolescents my colleagues and I treat have generally been given a wide variety of clinical diagnoses. Most commonly, these include major depressive disorder, some type of anxiety disorder (generalized anxiety disorder, social phobia, post-traumatic stress disorder, or agoraphobia), oppositional defiant disorder, a substance use disorder, and borderline personality disorder. There are many other possible diagnoses, but these are the ones that have been given to most of our kids at some point before we begin our work with them.

In the interest of full transparency, and this might sound strange to some, in IFFT we tend not to think much about the child's diagnosis (or more commonly, diagnoses plural, as most kids have picked up two, three, four, or more along the way). This might sound a bit odd, and it goes against the grain of my profession somewhat, but honestly it's not as important as one might think. Of course, if a teen is showing symptoms of depressed mood, social anxiety, substance use, or what have you, trust me we're all over it. We treat whatever the presenting problems are, using whatever treatment approach or method that meets the standard of care for those presenting problems. For example, if an adolescent has been diagnosed with borderline personality disorder, a disorder characterized by high emotional reactivity, unstable relationships, and often self-harm, we are for sure going to be incorporating dialectical behavior therapy in that person's treatment (much more on DBT in the next chapter). Or, if a child is socially phobic (an avoidance of social situations that make them anxious), we would use exposure therapy. Exposure is a well-established treatment for anxiety disorders, and it involves carefully sending the child into increasingly challenging social situations until those situations are no longer anxiety-producing.

DOI: 10.4324/9781003397366-7

So, IFFT is transdiagnostic, meaning we work with a great deal of pre-senting problems, but rather than focus on "disorders," these are the two broad clusters of presenting problems and symptoms that we typically treat:

- Suicidal and self-harming. Suicidal kids who talk about wanting to be dead and who might try to take their own lives. Self-harm is not about wanting to be dead, but it's about cutting or burning themselves, and on occasion might include behaviors that are even more extreme (like swallowing glass or other sharp objects). Typically, self-harm occurs in response to an upset of some kind, such as conflict with a parent or peer. Children and teens who hurt themselves are often placed into psychi-atric hospitals and/or a residential treatment program, sometimes many, many times before we see them. Chapters 6 and 7 focus on this type of problem, as well as the steps involved in successfully treating it, along with an actual case example in Chapter 8.
- Anxious and avoidant. Children and teens with a great deal of anxiety often become very avoidant and socially isolated. They tend to avoid the stuff of life—going to school, interacting with family, leaving their bedroom, and often don't bathe or take care of their personal hygiene. Avoidant kids can be very frustrating to parents because they can easily defeat any of the parents' attempts to get them to re-engage in life. These kids can be suicidal too, but not always. The avoidant behavior often comes with a strong oppositional component ("You can't make me take a shower"). We'll talk in much more detail about anxious/avoidant patients in Chapters 9 and 10, and along with a case example in Chapter 11.

It seems to me that many of the diagnoses given to children and adolescents can be subsumed under these two broad categories of presenting problems. And, of course, these are not always neatly defined, discrete categories; a child can be anxiously avoidant also be suicidal at the same time. For ex-ample, post-traumatic stress disorder, an anxiety disorder that results after exposure to one or more traumatic events that can lead to emotional reactivity and hypervigilance (scanning the environment for danger), can sometimes include self-harm and avoidance (Yehuda et al., 2015). Similarly, major depressive disorder can lead to suicidal thoughts, social isolation, and irritability and anger. Throughout this book, we are going to be talking about how IFFT treats both of these broad categories and various inter-ventions and techniques that are highly effective for each one.

The Underlying Assumptions That Drive IFFT

As I mentioned previously, when a family brings in a child or teen for treatment, we begin with the assumption that there is nothing inherently "wrong" with them. Of course, there is most definitely something wrong in the child or teen's life, or the family would not be sitting in front of us in the first place. In truth, many things have gone very wrong, and it's our job to figure out what those things are and then mitigate or *disrupt* any contributing factors or influences that are playing a role in the child and family's problematic thoughts, feelings, and behavior.

In IFFT, we see families and treatment in a pretty straightforward way: solve enough problems and the kid gets better, fail to solve enough problems and the kid stays the same and maybe even gets worse.

Before we can fully unpack the structure of IFFT, we're going to need to talk about the underlying assumptions that drive the treatment. What are the things that IFFT therapists believe to be true—the theoretical lens through which we see children and their families? How we see that world matters a lot because it informs much of what we do to best help a struggling family.

The Role of Temperament in Children's Mental illness

One thing that became almost immediately apparent to me when I started working with families is that there is usually only one child or teen that the parents bring in for treatment, even though they often have other children who, in most cases, are more or less "normal." By normal, I mean they don't have a mental health condition and they lead fairly age-typical lives. How can this be so? Same parents and raised more or less in the same environment, however, this kid is off the rails but the siblings are fine.

The only possible explanation I can think of is that there is just something temperamentally different about the child or teen in treatment. Temperament has been defined as innate individual differences in emotional and behavioral tendencies that appear during infancy and are relatively stable over time and in various contexts and situations (Clauss et al., 2015). Think of the word "personality" as shorthand for temperament. If a parent describes their child as "emotionally sensitive" at present, there's a pretty good chance they'll say the child has "always been like that." This is also very true for strong-willed, oppositional children ("When they were toddlers, they were much more stubborn than their siblings.").

Temperament interacts with the environment to predict risk for mental and behavioral problems. Infants with "difficult" temperaments are characterized by high reactivity or strong responses to novel stimuli that place them at greater risk for behavioral difficulties and later childhood mental and behavioral issues (Derauf et al., 2011). Along these same lines, an "inhibited temperament" is a risk factor for developing mental illness. Inhibited temperament is the tendency to avoid new people, objects, and experiences. In one study, it was found that 43% of inhibited children developed social anxiety disorder by adolescence, compared with about one in 10 children who were not inhibited (Clauss et al., 2015).

Here's what I tell parents: *you've got a hard kid.* They very likely came into the world that way and are just much more difficult to parent than an average child or teenager (their siblings, for example). Some parents seem to have an intuitive understanding of this already ("Thank God we had more than one or we'd think we were terrible parents"). Amen to that. More commonly, however, parents blame themselves for their child's problems, and there is often a tremendous amount of guilt and shame that goes along with that belief. Our broader culture feeds into this narrative, as most people assume that when a child is struggling in some way it's probably because the parents are at fault.

In IFFT, we do not see parents as the cause of their child's problems, far from it. Of course, if a parent is physically, sexually, or emotionally abusive, then yes, that causes terrible psychological damage to children. While these types of parents absolutely exist, they are, by far, not most parents. Most parents in my experience are kind-hearted, loving people who are doing their best but have no idea how they got into this terrible situation and certainly no idea how to get out.

They are mystified as to why what they're doing works great with the child's siblings but absolutely does not work with the child in treatment. Again, it is very likely they're just a more difficult-to-parent kid. I tell parents that if they took their child out of their own family and plopped them into another random family, the kid would very likely be off the rails there too. Plop them into an abusive family? Watch out—things would be far, far worse. I also tell parents that I can't change the child's temperament; that is, I cannot turn this human being into an entirely different human being, but I can, for sure, intervene in countless ways to make their situation far better than it is currently.

And I'd be remiss if I didn't say that the parents' temperaments didn't come into play as well. Some parents are just more relaxed and even-tempered (generally a good trait when it comes to parenting), whereas others naturally run hotter and are more reactive (not such a good trait when raising a very sensitive or strong-willed child).

So, okay, you've got a hard kid. How do we make that work? So much of my job entails helping parents get into a better rhythm with their child, how to peacefully co-exist with a difficult kid, and most importantly, how to have the best possible relationship with them, now and forever. I strongly believe that in many instances we do not get the kids we expected to have; we get the ones we actually have. We have plans for them, darn it: valedictorian, Harvard, and Nobel-prize winner, but shoot—turns out these unique, living, breathing, three-dimensional creatures have plans of their own. So if you believe that family and relationships are the things that really count the most in life, it's good to figure out how to best love and cherish the kid you actually have rather than the one you expected to have.

Okay, so temperament plays a role in the development of child's mental health problems, but there's much more to the story than just that.

Bidirectional Mutual Influences

In IFFT, we believe strongly that children and adolescents are in a constant state of bidirectional mutual influence with others in their social environment. The things the child does and says affect the things that others do and say in return. This notion was first proposed by Robert Bell (1968) when he argued that a child's behavior is not just a result of their parents' influence, but that the parents' behavior is equally influenced by the child's behavior. As parents, we believe that the ways in which we interact with our children influence their behavior in a hopefully positive direction. This is true, but it is equally true that the ways our children interact with us influence our behavior in return. This bidirectional mutual influence in many cases is a very positive thing: a parent who is playful and engaged with their child is very likely going to elicit playful behavior from the child in return, which then provides that parent with the incentive to be playful more often, and so on. Bidirectional mutual influence occurs not just between parents and their children, but it occurs in all human relationships. Every interaction we have with another person is an opportunity to influence that person, and their responses in return are opportunities to influence us.

However, there is a dark side to all of this too. Bidirectional influence can also unfold in very unhelpful ways that are highly relevant to children with mental health challenges.

Positive and Negative "Resonance"

Children and adolescents, especially those with challenging behavior, can and often do influence their parents' behavior in undesirable ways. Even very good, well-intentioned parents can often fall into problematic behavior patterns in response to their child's challenging behavior. This, in turn, has the effect of worsening the child's behavior, thereby resulting in less effective and even more unhelpful parenting, and so on. This moment-by-moment "resonance," or feedback loop between family members occurs without their awareness (unconsciously) but gets repeated over and over, and grows more firmly entrenched within families over time.

A *negative resonant exchange* is one that mutually and progressively worsens both the parent and the child's interactions. This often results in high emotional arousal (usually anger) on both sides, leading to conflict situations that play out repeatedly over time. In contrast, a *positive resonant exchange*—one that results in warmth, empathy, and connection—becomes increasingly rare in the family. Here's what it boils down to: negative resonant exchanges amplify the child's problematic behavior, and positive resonant exchanges reduce or mitigate a child's problematic behavior.

Negative resonant exchanges, such as heated arguments, criticism, or stonewalling (minimally engaging as a passive way to convey anger) have a profoundly corrosive effect on relationships within the family. Both the parents and the child become angry and frustrated with each other, again and again, building up entrenched resentments. Day-to-day interactions become very strained, and the ratio of positive interactions to negative interactions becomes very far off balance, and problems just continue to get worse and worse. One teenage patient described it this way: "It's like everyone's claws are out all of the time, ready to scratch at any moment."

Here's a simple but very common example—one that includes elements of both temperament and bidirectionality. Let's say a parent is raising an unusually strong-willed teenager, which, as I mentioned, is going to make them harder to parent than the average kid. They just have a tendency to say "no" far more often and tend to become much more oppositional if they feel challenged or controlled in any way. Now let's add three more variables to the equation: this particular kid is not a super strong student, neither are they especially motivated to do well in school (two characteristics that tend to go hand in hand), but the parents believe grades are very important. For most families in this type of situation, homework and grades are a flashpoint, a regular source of conflict, upset, and bad feelings.

Most parents are reasonable at first—they start off by just telling the kid to do their homework and try to get caught up. The kid in return, as most do in this scenario, says "Okay." Whether they mean it or not, who knows, but most will say that if for no other reason than to get their parents off their back and bring the conversation to a close.

So far, so good.

A little time goes by and the parents check again and find even more missing assignments. Now they're mad, hotter, and not so nice about it. In the language of video games, the parents have leveled up. They become way more insistent and commanding, with "Get your homework done now! I'm not going to tell you again." The kid does the same thing in return—leveling up, too, by getting equally mad and becoming even more stubborn. This dynamic illustrates two concepts that I have mentioned already: *mirroring and matching* and a *tug-of-war*, making everyone's behavior progressively worse. The word I use to describe this is *pinging;* each one is pinging off the other. What began as a discussion (well, sort of) about homework is now unmistakably a full-on argument, which in most cases leaves everyone feeling angry, frustrated, and pretty certain they weren't the one at fault and the other person was. And, obviously, no homework gets done.

Now, of course, in almost all families there can be arguments about just about anything. However, in reasonably high-functioning families, exchanges like this only spin out occasionally, and it's not a big deal, so they can shake it off and recover from it easily. However, if this scene, or other versions of it, repeats itself over and over, now you're going to have some serious problems. Family members start getting resentful of one another, hold grudges, and assume the worst of each other. This increases the probability of more negative resonance, that is, decreased warmth, and increased anger and disconnection. There's also a very good chance that someone is going to diagnose this teenager with oppositional defiant disorder, which seems entirely unfair to me. This teen is strong-willed and stubborn, sure, but I cannot in good conscious label them with a "disorder," given that this is clearly, in part, a family dynamic issue.

Bidirectional Resonance Within Other Important Subsystems: Siblings, Peers, and School

Bidirectional influences don't exist just between the parent and the child or adolescent. Other social influences are present in the child's life that can also create either positive or negative resonance. This, in turn, can either further amplify or reduce the child's problematic behaviors. In addition to the bidirectional influence that occurs between parent and child, bidirectional influences also exist between the child and three other important relational subsystems: siblings, peers, and school. Social, and contextual variables in these other areas play a vital role in the child's well-being, day-to-day behavior, and overall functioning. All components of each of the five relational subsystems (the child's temperament, parents, siblings, peers, and school) interact with each other to create feedback loops, which can have an impact on the child's mental health condition for better or worse (Figure 5.1).

The interplay between each of the five subsystems can be enormously complex. For example, a child or teen who is temperamentally strong-willed and/or emotionally reactive will be less inclined to follow rules. This type of behavior at home is likely to trigger a less-than-ideal response from the parents, who typically respond by becoming increasingly strict and inflexible. The child will respond to these efforts at control with anger and more rule-breaking behavior. Their easier-to-parent siblings will almost certainly have less conflict with the parents, resulting in a more gentle style of parenting. The harder kid notices this preferential treatment ("You treat them differently and it's not fair"), which causes even more resentment and rule-breaking behavior. The child will start to pull away from

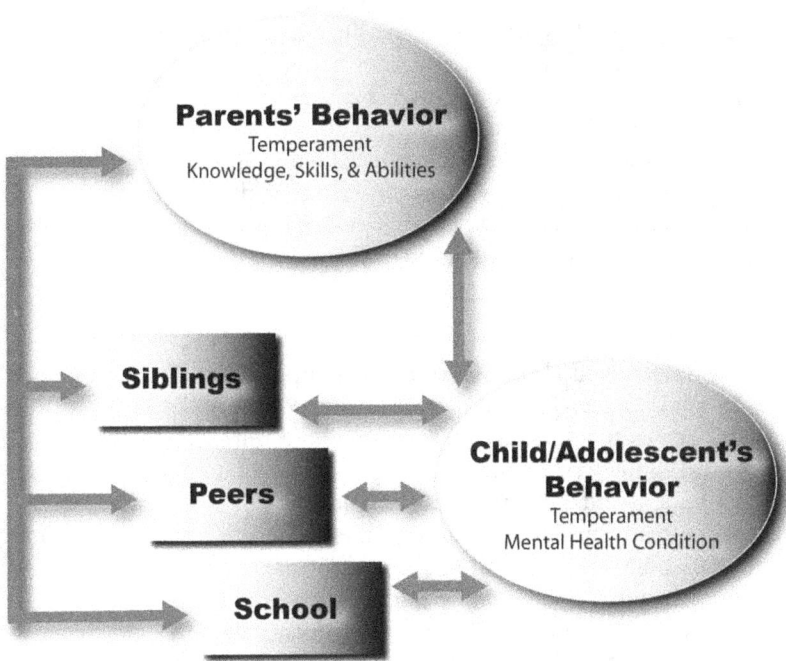

Figure 5.1 Bidirectional mutual influence between the child and the four relational subsystems.

their family and siblings, feeling increasingly disconnected and an outsider in their own home.

At school, the child's rule-breaking behavior, fueled by resentment at home, results in conflict with teachers and, likely, very little work completion. This becomes known to the parents and they respond by imposing even stricter, more rigid discipline at home. To further complicate the matter, the child's teachers will also respond to the rule-breaking behavior by adopting stronger disciplinary measures of their own that are visible to the other students. Research has shown that this dynamic in the classroom, especially when this bidirectional pattern between teacher and student occurs early in school, negatively affects the child's peer status (L'Écuyer et al., 2021). Criticism and negative attention from a teacher typically results in the more positive, prosocial peers pulling away, and so the child will likely gravitate to peers who encourage and reinforce more rule-breaking behavior, which becomes an extremely powerful influence in their lives.

Negative peer influences are, in my experience, the single most important driving factor in a child's mental health condition, especially for adolescents. Psychologist Judith Rich Harris caused quite an upset in the field of developmental psychology when she argued very convincingly that by the time a child is an adolescent, they are far more influenced by the behavior of their friend group than by their parents (Harris, 2009). Similarly, Thomas Dishion and his colleagues (1999) described what he refers to as "deviance training." When teens with rule-breaking tendencies are put together in groups with other rule-breaking teens, they subtly reinforce each other's negative behavior through praise and approval and fail to reinforce positive, prosocial behavior.

Situational Influences

So far, we have talked about the role that temperament and bidirectional influences play in the onset and maintenance of a child's mental health condition. Let us turn our attention now to the third major contributor: the powerful influence of situations to greatly affect a child's well-being.

In Chapters 1 and 2, I spoke about some of the leading factors that appear to be contributing to a surge in mental health problems in young people, including social isolation, the impact of smartphones and social media, suggestibility, social/emotional/behavioral contagion, and so on. In IFFT, we look at these as situational influences, defined as any social or environmental factor that is contributing to the child's mental health condition. At the start of treatment with every family, we are on the hunt to identify and then neutralize or at least mitigate any situational influences that we think are playing a role in the child's problematic thoughts, feelings, and behavior.

There has been quite a bit of research done by social psychologists that sheds light on the power of the situation to affect how we think and what we do. Most of us tend to believe we have a relatively steady "self," or a predictable, consistent personality and set of behaviors that can be counted on over time and across situations. This is likely true to some degree, but research suggests that human behavior can be highly situationally dependent. We are often quite surprised when a person behaves in a way that seems truly out of character, such as a formerly loyal spouse who is unfaithful, a person who is typically a rule-follower who cheats on their taxes, or a favorite Hollywood celebrity accused of sexual misconduct. ("I never would have guessed they were capable of that. They seem so nice.")

A great illustration of this comes from what is known as the Good Samaritan Study conducted in the early 1970s by John Darley and David Batson (1973). They decided to study helping behavior in a group of people likely to be reasonably selfless and compassionate: seminary students training to become priests. Sixty-seven participants in the study were asked to deliver a sermon on the parable of the Good Samaritan, which is about helping others in need. The subjects were randomly assigned to two conditions: the hurried condition, in which they were asked to go across campus to deliver the sermon but were told they were running late and needed to hurry, and an unhurried condition in which the subjects were told they had plenty of time to get there. The students then walked alone following the same path to the building where they would deliver the sermon. On the way there, each encountered a staged scene of a person slumped in a doorway with his eyes closed, coughing and moaning. And what did the experimenters find? Only 10% of the seminary students in the hurried condition stopped to help the person, whereas 63% of the students in the unhurried condition stopped. It is important to note again that these are *seminary students*, whose behavior became highly uncharacteristic simply because they were in a hurry. Change the situation, change the person. (Even more sadly perhaps, note that in the unhurried condition, 37% of the students still did not stop to help.)

This study, and variations on it, has been replicated many times and the findings are clear: how we think we're going to behave in a situation often largely depends on the situation itself, especially if that situation is novel or unfamiliar. If you are interested in learning more about this fascinating aspect of human nature, Lee Ross and Richard Nisbitt (1991) unpack it fully in their work, *The Person and the Situation: Perspectives of Social Psychology*.

Why does this matter? Because in IFFT, we assume that the child's thoughts, feelings, and behaviors are largely influenced by the current set of situational variables (their circumstances) in which they find themselves. Parents often say to me, "We don't know our own child anymore" because in many respects the child's current behavior is so vastly different from what it was in years past. Is the kid different? I don't think so, but the circumstances are now very different. I would argue that by and large, all of our young patients are good kids who now find themselves in bad situations, and they are behaving as just about anyone would in the same set of circumstances. They have no idea how they got there, no idea what's making them this way, and certainly no idea of how to get themselves out.

Our job as clinicians is to identify and, most importantly, *disrupt* as many situational variables as we can that are having a negative impact on the child's well-being. For example, what if a teenager is spending, many, many hours a day on a device? *Disrupt*. If there are barriers getting in the way of doing homework? *Disrupt*. If the teen goes out and gets high with other teens? *Disrupt*. If a parent gets frustrated and loses their temper? *Disrupt*. If the child has no friends because they are socially avoidant? *Disrupt*. There are countless other examples of situational variables like these, and later in the book I'll be teaching you how to disrupt them.

IFFT in a Nutshell

As we've learned, IFFT is based on the premise that childhood mental illness can be best understood and treated within the social context in which the child resides, especially, but not limited to, their family. IFFT does not view "mental illness" as localized solely within the child; remember, it's a family problem to solve. Instead, the current problems are based on the complex interplay that exists between the child's difficult-to-parent temperament, bidirectional mutual influences with others, and the negative situational variables that exist, which play a role in the child's day-to-day life and overall functioning.

IFFT views family as the single best, most effective mechanism of change, far more so than we, the treatment providers are. Our role is simply to act as catalysts, as facilitators, to positively impact the family system, which in turn positively impacts the child's mental health condition.

In short, families are medicine.

IFFT is, in part, a behavior-based treatment that is highly focused on the reduction of problematic behavior in the child or adolescent. In just about every family we treat, parents simply do not know what to do in the face of such challenging behavior. Parenting strategies that generally work quite well for less difficult-to-parent kids are simply not effective, and so IFFT places a heavy emphasis very early in treatment on teaching parents how to reduce problematic behavior. It's the child's behavior—such as threats of suicide and self-harm, disrespect, breaking rules, damaging property, running away, verbal and sometimes physical aggression, school refusal, screen addiction, and so on—that brings them into treatment in the first place. I would be a terrible therapist if, week after week, I kept seeing a family and I hadn't been able to improve the child's behavior. IFFT uses very specialized, focused, targeted behavioral interventions that are generally unknown to most parents, and we begin reducing problematic behavior from the very first session. This, in turn, significantly reduces family distress and makes it possible for everyone to work on improving connection, communication, and collaborative problem-solving, and ultimately create stronger attachments.

At its core, IFFT seeks to assess, understand, and most importantly *disrupt* patterns and sources of negative bidirectional and situational influences. If done successfully, the net result of these efforts is a reduction in a child or teen's mental health symptoms, as well as a significant improvement in their overall functioning and well-being. Again, solve enough problems and the kid gets better.

Here are some questions we try to answer when a family first presents for treatment. What is the child's temperament and how does it affect the parents' behavior in response? How do the parents typically respond in the face of challenging behavior? That is, do they stay reasonably calm and matter-of-fact, or do they sometimes get angry and reactive? What skills do we think they need to more effectively parent a child who can often be difficult and strong-willed or emotionally reactive? How does the child's behavior influence the behavior of siblings, and vice versa, and how can these problematic interactions be successfully mitigated? What is the nature of the child's academic experience and the quality of their relationship with teachers? How can school-related problems (not doing homework, getting suspended, etc.) be effectively addressed so as to reduce conflict at home? What is the nature of the child's peer group—are they a source of support and positive modeling or do they influence the child's behavior in a negative direction? What role are devices and social media playing in all of this—how much time is the child spending on devices, who are they communicating with, and what is being said? What skills can we teach the child to better navigate negative peer influences or connect them to a more positive, pro-social peer group? And many, many more questions like these.

I think of family treatment in general, and behavior in particular, very much like a mathematical equation. The answers to these, and other questions, become variables in the equation that fall to the left of the equals sign, with the child's overall functioning at this moment to the right of it. For example, consider one example: Variable 1 (V1; the child's temperament); V2 parents' current skill set; V3 the presence of negative peer influences; V4 current degree of closeness and connection in the home; V5 amount of reactivity in the home; V6 negative school influences; V7 excessive time on devices; V8 the crowding out effect of that time on devices; V9 who the child is communicating with on those devices; and V10 the degree of social isolation present. So, with this particular kid, it looks like:

$$V1 + V2 + V3 + V4 + V5 + V6 + V7 + V8 + V9 + V10$$
$$= \text{Child's overall functioning}$$

When you think of it this way for the first time, it should become clear that there are 10 possible points of clinical intervention within this particular family (sometimes there are more points of intervention than this family, sometimes less). Each of these variables is an opportunity for the clinician to effect positive change, which might include: creating a structure to reduce screen time; monitoring online activity; teaching more effective communication and problem-solving skills; introducing incentives to engage in other wellness-enhancing activities (spending time with family, getting some exercise; implementing strategies to entice that child out of their bedroom; creating opportunities for the child to come into contact with more positive peers; and so on. Any variable in the equation, when improved, will likely also result in improvement in the child's overall functioning and mental health. This is the essence of IFFT: *What situational variables are negatively impacting the child, what situational variables can we change, and what strategies are going to be most effective in bringing about these changes?*

Back to diagnosis for a moment. On some occasions, we are able to quickly intervene and modify enough of these variables so that within just a few months there is pretty substantial behavioral, emotional, and functional improvement. If this was a case of major depressive disorder, or some sort of biologically-based mental illness, how did that happen so fast? Change the situation, change the kid.

Interestingly, we've also learned that when all of the variables in the equation remain constant, the child's overall functioning also remains constant. So, if you can change enough of these variables, and to a sufficient degree, the child's functioning not only improves but remains stable and positive over time.

This entire book is about changing variables in the equation.

IFFT is a Team-Based Approach

IFFT is a team-based, outpatient model consisting typically of three fully licensed therapists working with the family, with each clinician serving a very specific role and function. Almost all of the children and adolescents with whom we work have already received extensive outpatient therapy, and sometimes treatment delivered in more restrictive settings, such as psychiatric hospitals and residential treatment programs. However, despite these interventions, they still haven't gotten any better. As you might guess, these patients are extremely complex and present with behavior that is extraordinarily challenging. The probability of finding a single therapist with the necessary knowledge, skills, and abilities to effectively treat a family with a high-risk/high-needs child seems quite low to me.

I strongly believe that this is simply not a one-person job. Teams have the advantage of being diverse and heterogeneous, with each team member bringing their own unique skill set required to work with children and families with complex needs. Heterogeneous groups (mixed backgrounds and skill sets) demonstrate more creativity and make better decisions (Zaidi et al., 2010). One clinician might be strong in the area of behavior change strategies, while another is really good at cognitive behavioral therapy or dialectical behavioral therapy, or perhaps a more attachment-based approach. In IFFT, each team member relies on the skill set of the other therapists on the team. As is the case with adults in therapy, we've also found that children and teens can sometimes naturally connect better with one therapist over another. If the fit is not good for whatever reason, we can easily replace one team member with another, or the best-connected team member can assume the lead.

Here is one other very important point to understand about IFFT and the therapists who work with our families. *They are all very, very good.* I can say this with some confidence for several reasons. First, I feel strongly that given the complexities that our families present, they have a right to receive treatment from therapists with a demonstrated track record of competency. Being licensed is a good first step—it shows the person has accumulated the necessary number of supervised hours (about the equivalent of seeing patients full-time for two years) and has passed one and sometimes two written exams as well. An unlicensed therapist is one who is currently still in training, working under the supervision of someone with a license. They might someday be very good but, for now, they are clearly still in learning mode.

There has been quite a bit of research conducted on how someone gets good at something. K. Anders Ericsson and his colleagues (1993) caused quite a stir, which is still the subject of some debate even now, but their conclusions can be summarized as follows. When we think of someone who is highly competent, a person who has reached an expert level of performance, we tend to believe that they are uniquely talented in some way. Ericsson agrees that innate talent or natural ability does play a role in expert competency, but to reach a level of expert status even very talented people must spend many, many hours practicing something to get good at it. You simply cannot acquire a complex set of skills without spending an awful lot of time engaged in practice. Ericsson argues it's not just any kind of practice, it's what he refers to as deliberate practice, such as direct instruction from someone better at the skill than you; taking courses to acquire a deeper understanding of the skill; taking active steps to get better based on direct feedback; and of course the practicing itself. The number of practice hours that Ericsson arrived at to reach expert status is 10,000, the equivalent of a therapist in full-time practice for 10 years. Please do not take this as disrespect toward unlicensed or green therapists; I was one myself, obviously. I just feel strongly that the most challenging families with high-risk children and adolescents should be treated by experts, and not someone working their way in that direction.

Ericsson argues further that feedback plays a vital role in reaching high competency and expert status. Such a mechanism must exist to know if what you're doing is correct; for example, a tennis coach giving you feedback on form, or a music teacher telling you the proper way to hold your instrument. In IFFT, we regularly solicit feedback from our parents and their child or teen by asking them to complete a survey and rating us on warmth, empathy, ability to listen before intervening, how helpful the sessions are, and their overall satisfaction with treatment. This feedback allows us to make course corrections with the goal of improving our scores over time. In addition, we ask parents to complete a written daily log that summarizes both positive and negative events each day and to provide a numerical score that describes the day overall. This day-to-day feedback gives us a pretty good idea of whether we're on track, as well as which interventions worked and which ones didn't.

Frequency and Length of Treatment

Four one-hour therapy sessions are provided each week at the start of treatment, either in the home, the office, or remotely: individual therapy for the child, family therapy (the child and their parents together), parent therapy, and a 1:1 skills coach for the child. (If someone from an insurance company is reading this, these are outpatient CPT codes 90837, 90846, and 90847.) Out of necessity, every therapist in the world got good at doing telehealth sessions during COVID, and we found, surprisingly, that many kids (but not all) do just fine with remote sessions.

Sessions are faded (become less frequent) as the family stabilizes and the child's behavior improves, which typically occurs somewhere around the six-month mark of treatment. The total duration of services for most families is approximately nine months. IFFT, therefore, is not a quick treatment; if we knew how to do it faster we would, but we can't. We also feel strongly that demonstrated stability over time is really important—we need enough time to create new habits and make sure all of the variables in the equation remain constant (which means, again, that the child's functioning will remain constant once we back out).

In IFFT, the individual therapist and family therapist is the same clinician because, truthfully, as I've already mentioned, family therapy can be very hard, both for the family and the clinician. We have found it to be essential that the child or teen has a close, trusting relationship with the family therapist. As family therapy can be challenging (we're often talking about some very difficult topics), the family therapist often relies on the strong relationship that has been built in the individual sessions.

We are going to get much deeper into session content, but, for now, here's an overview of each of the four weekly sessions.

Individual therapy most often follows a cognitive behavioral therapy (CBT) approach and/or the use of dialectical behavior therapy (DBT) (Beck, 2011; Linehan, 1993). We'll talk much more about these approaches in just a bit. They are well-established treatment models that are variations on helping a person become aware of, and change, unhelpful thinking patterns that can lead to negative feelings and problematic behavior. However, there are very few therapists who follow just one approach, and that includes IFFT as well. Therapy is a fast-moving, fluid, often complicated process, and I find myself moving through multiple techniques and strategies, sometimes dozens of them in a single session.

Family therapy typically attempts to build on positive experiences within the family (what's working and going well), balanced with discussions and resolutions of past and present problem events, all with the goal of building stronger connection and attachment. As I mentioned, family therapy is probably the most difficult of the four sessions. Parents often have so much pent-up frustration and anger that they want to dump it all out in the first session, which obviously is not a good idea. Most of our parents have not done much family therapy before they come to us, so we spend a lot of time orienting them to the process and putting some structure in place— otherwise, all hell would break loose. We've found as well that kids have a lot of misconceptions and sometimes anxiety around family therapy because they assume they are the problem and they're just going to be hammered by their parents and the therapist for the entire hour. To mitigate this, we always start and end sessions on what has occurred during the week that's positive, with a problem area sandwiched in between.

In IFFT, all family therapy sessions are either video- or audio-recorded with the full consent of the parents and the child or teen (but we never record the child's individual sessions). Those sessions are reviewed by me and by other team members for several important reasons. Sometimes when a therapist is right in the middle of it, things in session might go by unnoticed, but they may be easier for another set of eyes to spot. Back to the notion of the importance of a team model: other team members can sometimes offer suggestions or alternatives, particularly if the family therapist gets stuck in some way.

The 1:1 skills coach works directly with the child or teen, and primarily (but not exclusively) focuses on DBT skills (emotion regulation, distress tolerance, interpersonal effectiveness, and mindfulness) (Linehan & Wilks, 2015). Rather than tell kids what not to do, it's generally a far better idea to teach them what they can do differently instead, in order to achieve their preferred outcome ("You know I've found negotiating with someone makes it far more likely I'll get what I want. I'm an excellent negotiator in fact. Can I show you what that might look like with your parents?").

Parent therapy, the fourth and final session each week, focuses on im- proving several key areas within the family. First, there is an emphasis on improving family functioning, which has the effect of mitigating the severity of a child's mental illness. It reduces reactivity in the family and improves communication skills; develops collaborative problem-solving skills, inter- vening more effectively on problematic behavior; and increases attentiveness, warmth, and connection. As I've mentioned previously, there is also a heavy emphasis in parent therapy on teaching parents behavior change strategies that work. Most of these strategies are largely unknown to parents, and some are quite sophisticated (but easy enough to learn).

I believe it is now time to do a deep dive into treating the two most commonly presenting problems we see in our clinic: self-harming/suicidal behaviors and anxious avoidance.

Chief Takeaways from Chapter 5

For Parents

- Don't get too stuck on your child or teen's diagnosis. Definitely try to understand it, of course, but it's a better use of time and energy to focus instead on what to do about it.
- If your child is struggling with a serious mental health challenge, they likely have a more difficult-to-parent temperament (personality). They didn't ask to be this way; they just are. They're going to be harder to raise than the average kid and that's okay.
- You influence your child's behavior just as much as they influence yours. We change another person's behavior by first changing our own.
- Much of what's going on with your child has to do with the situational influences that are affecting their mental health (peers, devices, and so on). They're a good kid stuck in a bad set of circumstances, most of which have nothing to do with you. But, you're the only person who can make their situation better.
- One therapist can't do it all, no matter how good they are. And, if you're looking for a therapist, try to find someone who's been doing it for about 10 years or longer if you can.

For Clinicians

- Maybe consider focusing a bit less on diagnosis and more on mitigating situational variables that are influencing the child or teen to demonstrate those symptoms.
- Be on the lookout for fixed patterns of communication or interactions that leave everyone in the family feeling bad and try to change them (and have them practice what works better).
- Try to consider as many situational variables as you can, and look for ways you or the parents can mitigate and neutralize those influences. Change the situation and you'll change the kid.
- Consider a team-based approach if you're not already doing so. It's good to have another set of eyes on challenging cases, and it makes the job easier and your work more effective.
- Family therapy is hard, so buckle up. But you have my utmost gratitude and admiration for doing it.

Bonus Tip for Insurance Companies

- Effective family therapy for serious childhood mental illness can be delivered very effectively on an outpatient basis using CPT codes 90837, 90846, and 90837.

References

Beck, J. S. (2011). *Cognitive behavior therapy: Basics and beyond* (2nd ed.). Guilford Press.

Bell, R. Q. (1968). A reinterpretation of the direction of effects in studies of socialization. *Psychological Review*, *75*(2), 81–95. 10.1037/h0025583

Clauss, J. A., Avery, S. N., & Blackford, J. U. (2015). The nature of individual differences in inhibited temperament and risk for psychiatric disease: A review and meta-analysis. *Progress in Neurobiology*, *127*, 23–45. 10.1016/j.pneurobio.2015. 03.001

Darley, J. M., & Batson, C. D. (1973). "From Jerusalem to Jericho": A study of situational and dispositional variables in helping behavior. *Journal of Personality and Social Psychology*, *27*(1), 100–108. 10.1037/h0034449

Derauf, C., LaGasse, L., Smith, L., Newman, E., Shah, R., Arria, A., Huestis, M., Haning, W., Strauss, A., Della Grotta, S., Dansereau, L., Lin, H., & Lester, B. (2011). Infant temperament and high risk environment relate to behavior problems and language in toddlers. *Journal of Developmental & Behavioral Pediatrics*, *32*(2), 125–135. 10.1097/DBP.0b013e31820839d7

Dishion, T. J., McCord, J., & Poulin, F. (1999). When interventions harm: Peer groups and problem behavior. *American Psychologist*, *54*(9), 755–764. 10.103 7/0003-066X.54.9.755

Ericsson, K. A., Krampe, R. T., & Tesch-Römer, C. (1993). The role of deliberate practice in the acquisition of expert performance. *Psychological Review*, *100*(3), 363–406. 10.1037/0033-295X.100.3.363

Harris, J. R. (2009). *The nurture assumption: Why children turn out the way they do*. Free Press.

L'Écuyer, R., Poulin, F., Vitaro, F., & Capuano, F. (2021). Bidirectional links between teachers' disciplinary practices, students' peer status, and students' aggression in kindergarten. *Research on Child and Adolescent Psychopathology*, *9*(5), 671–682. 10.1007/s10802-021-00767-3

Linehan, M. M. (1993). *Cognitive-behavioral treatment of borderline personality disorder*. Guilford Press.

Linehan, M. M., & Wilks, C. R. (2015). The course and evolution of dialectical behavior therapy. *American Journal of Psychotherapy*, *69*(2), 97–110. 10.1176/ appi.psychotherapy.2015.69.2.97

Ross, L., & Nisbett, R. E. (1991). *The person and the situation: Perspectives of social psychology*. McGraw-Hill Book Company.

Yehuda, R., Hoge, C. W., McFarlane, A. C., Vermetten, E., Lanius, R. A., Nievergelt, C. M., Hobfoll, S. E., Koenen, K. C., Neylan, T. C., & Hyman, S. E. (2015). Post-traumatic stress disorder. *Nature Reviews Disease Primers, 1,* Article 15057. 10.1038/nrdp.2015.57

Zaidi, S. M. A., Saif, M. I., & Zaheer, A. (2010). The effect of workgroup heterogeneity on decision making: An empirical investigation. *African Journal of Business Management, 4*(10), 2132–2139.

Part II

Treating Suicide and Self-Harm

6 Suicide and Self-Harm

Prevalence, Evidence-Based Treatments, and the Role of Family and Situations

> *"Maricela," a 13-year-old girl diagnosed with major depressive disorder and a history of self-harm (cutting) and one overdose attempt, is alone in her room in the dark. As is often the case, she has been angry and withdrawn all day. Her mother is worried, so she goes into Maricela's room and notices that she is curled up on her bed wearing a long-sleeved sweatshirt despite the warm weather. Her mother knows what this probably means—Maricela has cut again. Her mother asks if she is okay, but Maricela screams at her and tells her to get out of her room. How the family responds in the next few minutes is going to determine whether they can get through this event successfully, or if it's going to escalate further and involve a trip to the emergency room and, perhaps, even a stay in a psychiatric hospital.*

Treating children and adolescents who hurt themselves is not for the faint of heart. The stakes are very high for everyone involved: The parents, the child or teen themselves, and the treating clinicians. For parents, the thought that their child could hurt themselves or take their own life at any moment is one of the most terrifying and heartbreaking situations they will ever likely encounter. Parents love their children desperately and fiercely, and the thought of losing a child is unimaginable. Protecting one's child is, after all, a parent's job. Feeling powerless to help or understand why their previously happy, loving child would contemplate suicide or self-harm is a source of tremendous pain and suffering.

For the treating clinician, working with suicidal children and adolescents can be nothing short of harrowing. The responsibility is enormous, and any misstep in treatment has the potential for catastrophe. As discussed in Chapter 3, the treatment for getting a child back on course often involves gently asking more of them (to go to school, spend less time in their rooms, less time on devices, more time with family members, and so on). Balancing safety with change is not a simple, straightforward task. As

DOI: 10.4324/9781003397366-9

a clinician, I have had countless mornings in which I've woken up wondering if my young patients have survived the night.

Self-harming behavior, thankfully, is usually quite treatable. In this chapter, we will begin by looking at the prevalence of suicide and self-harm. We will examine the two most well-established, evidence-based models of treatment for self-injurious behaviors. I will describe these treatments in some detail, both for the practicing therapist wishing to learn more and for the parent who may have heard about these treatments and is seeking to be better informed. Next, in the following chapter, I will provide a detailed, step-by-step family-focused approach to successfully treating children and adolescents who hurt themselves. Finally, I will pull back the curtain for parents and show you exactly what is said between child and therapist so that you can see our work in action.

Prevalence of Suicide

Tragically, suicide is the second leading cause of death among 10–14-year-olds and 25–34-year-olds in the United States, and the fourth leading cause of death among 15–29-year-olds globally (National Institute of Mental Health [NIMH], n.d.-b; World Health Organization, 2021). Depressed adolescents are at a significantly elevated risk of reporting suicidal ideation, planning, and attempts (Stewart et al., 2018). Among adolescents, rates of suicidal ideation (thoughts) range from 12–17%, and attempts range from 4–8% (Kann et al., 2014). Between 2000 and 2018, suicide deaths escalated by 35%, with the suicide rate at 14.5 per 100,000 people in 2018, the highest in more than 50 years.

Nonsuicidal Self-Injury

Nonsuicidal self-injury is harm that causes pain or injury but is not intended to cause death. However, self-harm is a risk factor for subsequent suicide. One study examined risk factors associated with suicide following an episode of self-harm and concluded that previous episodes of self-harm were associated with a higher risk of dying by suicide (Chan et al., 2016).

Prevalence of Nonsuicidal Self-Injury

A review of studies published from 2005–2011, reporting on nonsuicidal self-injury and self-harm among adolescents from around the world, found that approximately 18% of adolescents from the general community report engaging in nonsuicidal self-injury and self-harm, with similar rates across the globe (Muehlenkamp et al., 2012). Analyses suggest that the lifetime prevalence of nonsuicidal self-injury for the total population in the U.S. is approximately 6%, including just over 1% who reported having self-injured over 10 times. Lifetime prevalence was notably higher among those aged 30 years or younger at 19%, consistent with other figures in young adults (Whitlock et al., 2006).

Evidence-Based Models of Treatment

I am going into some detail here because I've learned that many parents hear about these two models of therapy, but the mental health community generally doesn't do a very good job of explaining what they are.

Cognitive Behavior Therapy

History

Cognitive behavior therapy (CBT) focuses on how thoughts, feelings, and behaviors influence one another (Beck Institute, n.d.-b). The basic idea of this approach is that our thoughts often become distorted and misleading, which then results in negative emotions. When combined together, distorted thoughts and negative feelings often lead to problematic behavior. Learning how to identify and evaluate our distorted thoughts can ultimately allow us to think more realistically, thereby changing how we feel and behave. CBT was developed by psychiatrist Aaron Beck as a way to help people recognize their negative thoughts and behaviors so that they can change them (Beck Institute, n.d.-a).

Treatment Components

CBT treatment typically endeavors to change both thinking and behavior (American Psychological Association [APA], 2017). According to the cognitive model, a situation can result in an individual having automatic thoughts, which then result in subsequent emotional, behavioral, and physiological responses. These automatic thoughts occur spontaneously, so much so that people may not immediately recognize them without practice. For example, negative automatic thoughts after failing an exam might include, "I'm so dumb" or "I'm a failure." These negative automatic thoughts can then result in emotional (e.g., sadness), behavioral (e.g., social withdrawal), and physiological responses (e.g., increased stress hormones) (Beck Institute, n.d.-b).

Noticing and challenging cognitive distortions is a key part of CBT. Listed below are examples of cognitive distortions, according to another psychiatrist David Burns, along with brief descriptions of each (Burns, 1980). *[Side note: I have found teaching my patients how to spot these 10 distortions in their thinking, and how to effectively challenge resultant negative thoughts, to be the single most useful thing I've ever learned.]*

All-Or-Nothing Thinking. The self and the world are looked at in absolute terms; there are no shades of gray. This leads to thinking in extremes. For example, during a self-injury relapse, one might tell themselves, "All that time in therapy is a waste of time; I'm no better at all."

Overgeneralization. One event is interpreted as part of an ongoing, neverending pattern. A patient might say, "I couldn't even get through this situation, so how can I handle life?"

Mental Filter. Negatives are brooded over while positives are ignored. People filter out every other piece of information, retaining only the negative.

Discounting the Positives. Positive things "don't count." A child or teen who engages in self-harm might not be thinking about all of the times they successfully resisted the urge to hurt themselves.

Jumping to Conclusions. "Mind reading" and "fortune telling" are two common ways a patient may jump to conclusions. Mind reading assumes you know the motives or intentions of another person, as though you could read their mind. For example, a teen might feel hurt because their best friend didn't respond right away to a text message, when in fact the friend was just doing their homework. Fortune telling predicts that events will turn out badly. The teen in the example above might predict that now they will lose all of their friends.

Magnification or Minimization. Things are either blown far out of proportion or their importance is reduced inappropriately. For someone struggling with suicidality, this might look like magnifying their perceived negative effects on others ("My friends must all hate me. I haven't heard from them in weeks."), while minimizing how people would react if they were to complete a suicide attempt ("People would be better off without me, it's not like I matter").

Emotional Reasoning. Reason comes from one's feelings rather than reality. For example, "I feel worthless, so I must be worthless."

"Should" Statements. "Should" or "Shouldn't" statements are used to criticize oneself or others (e.g., "I shouldn't have made a mistake"). Similar statements include "must," "ought," or "have to." For example, a child learning the violin might think "I should be able to play this song with no mistakes," and end up getting upset at themselves when they do make mistakes. *[Side note: The easiest way to neutralizee the negative power of a "should" is to replace it with "prefer." Nothing wrong with "I prefer that I had played this song with no mistakes."]*

Labeling. A type of overgeneralization in which the entire self or other is seen as the whole label. For example, instead of "I failed my math test," labeling distorts the thought into "I am a failure."

Personalization and Blame. A person blames themselves for something for which they were not at fault, or blames others for everything while one's own contributions to a problem are overlooked. For example, a child might blame themselves for their parents' divorce (personalization). The parents might blame one another for the failed marriage, instead of considering how they each contributed to the deterioration of the relationship (blame).

In CBT, the following strategies are used to challenge and restructure an automatic negative thought.

Identify the Distortion. Writing down one's negative thoughts makes it easier to see which cognitive distortions are at play, allowing the individual to consider the issue in a more realistic and fact-based light. The identification of even one distortion in the thought is a good indication that the thought probably should be challenged.

Examine the Evidence. Evidence for or against a negative thought is examined, rather than assuming the negative thought is true by default.

The Double-Standard Method. This involves talking to oneself in a compassionate rather than harsh manner, much like one would to a friend with a similar issue.

The Experimental Technique. The negative thought's validity is tested. The "experiment" would be relevant to the specific thought in question. For example, if the negative thought is "Everyone will think I'm disgusting when they see my self-harm scars," one might test this by intentionally showing their scars and observing people's reactions, if any.

The Survey Method. Asking other people questions allows the individual to evaluate whether their thoughts and attitudes are realistic.

Define Terms. Attempting to clearly define the labels given to oneself illuminates the fact that the label has no real definition.

Re-Attribution. This involves thinking more holistically about a problem and considering all the factors that may play a part, rather than assuming the individual is solely to blame.

It is worth noting that not all CBT will employ every strategy listed above (APA, 2017). Rather, these techniques may be thought of as a "toolbox" of skills the patient can apply whenever needed. Additionally, while the above techniques are well-known and often used in therapy, the list is by no means exhaustive.

Outcome Studies on CBT

CBT has strong empirical support that it is an effective treatment for chronically depressed adult patients, as well as adults with anxiety and related disorders (Leuzinger-Bohleber et al., 2019; Wootton et al., 2015). In a 2018 study, brief CBT led to consistently low rates of suicide attempts across patient severity (i.e., low, medium, or high suicide risk), whereas treatment as usual (something other than CBT) was associated with variable rates of suicidal behavior (Bryan et al., 2018). Moreover, research shows CBT is effective for treating children and adolescents with anxiety and depression, with analyses suggesting that outcomes may further improve when treatment includes behavioral activation, challenging thoughts, and caregivers' involvement (Seligman & Ollendick, 2011). CBT shows promise in treating children and adolescents struggling with suicidality and non-suicidal self-injury (Gilbert et al., 2020). CBT may also lead to notable improvements in alcohol and drug use problems, marital problems, eating disorders, and severe mental illness (APA, 2017).

My Own Take on Using CBT with Children and Adolescents Who Self-Harm

I find CBT to be a highly useful treatment when it becomes clear that a self-harm event was precipitated by an automatic negative thought that can be challenged and then restructured ("They made me mad so I cut myself."). CBT has become one of the mainstays of therapy—almost every therapist has received some training in it and makes an attempt at using it. However, I've learned that many therapists believe they're using CBT, but are actually using a watered-down or incomplete version of it. I find it takes a long time and a lot of practice to become highly skilled at CBT, and it's much harder to do than one might think. Lastly, CBT simply doesn't work for everyone, and to have it as your only clinical strategy when working with children and teens will likely result in less-than-ideal clinical outcomes.

Dialectical Behavior Therapy

History

Dialectical behavioral therapy (DBT) was developed by Marsha Linehan, PhD, and was initially used to treat highly suicidal patients who also met the diagnostic criteria for borderline personality disorder (BPD) (Linehan & Wilks, 2015). BPD severely affects one's ability to regulate emotions, which can lead to intense mood swings, an uncertain sense of self, unstable relationships, and impulsive self-destructive behavior (NIMH, n.d.-a). Dialectics refers to two or more seemingly contradictory concepts or viewpoints that in reality can occur at the same time. Thus, change and acceptance comprise the primary dialectic within DBT: Patients can be accepted just as they are, while the therapist simultaneously works to promote positive change and progress (Linehan & Wilks, 2015). *[Side note: Ask 10 therapists what dialectic means and all 10 of us will probably get it wrong. It's a tad confusing.]*

Treatment Components

In part, DBT consists of teaching patients four main skill modules: Mindfulness, distress tolerance, interpersonal effectiveness, and emotion regulation (Behavioral Tech, n.d.). Mindfulness and distress tolerance are acceptance-oriented, while interpersonal effectiveness and emotion regulation are change-oriented. Each skill category is described below with examples.

Mindfulness. Mindfulness means being completely present and aware of the moment. To be mindful is to be in the moment and experience it exactly as it is.

Distress Tolerance. Distress tolerance is the ability to withstand emotional pain in difficult situations, as opposed to changing or reducing that pain. This has to do with one's ability to sit with discomfort as it occurs, rather than reacting to it by engaging in self-harm.

Interpersonal Effectiveness. Interpersonal effectiveness is about maintaining respect for oneself and relationships with others and effectively asking for what one wants, while also being able to say no. Healthy boundaries are integral to building interpersonal effectiveness.

Emotion Regulation. Emotion regulation involves changing the emotions one wishes to change. This necessitates understanding how emotions work and building skills to manage emotions, instead of allowing emotions to manage the individual.

Outpatient (office) DBT consists of weekly or twice weekly individual therapy sessions, weekly skills training, and giving patients the ability to access their therapist after hours for in-the-moment coaching as needed.

DBT differs from CBT in its emphasis on dialectical thinking, acceptance, and mindfulness (Chapman, 2006). One might think of it as combining the cognitive aspects of CBT with Eastern mindfulness philosophies.

Nonlethal Self-Harm Versus Suicide

Linehan was the first to popularize the term *parasuicidal* behavior, which she defines as self-injury without the intention of taking one's life (Linehan et al., 1991). This is a very important concept because many adults and children who hurt themselves in some fashion (cutting is the most common) have no intention of ending their lives. The most common reason patients will give when asked why they hurt themselves is that it makes them feel better, likely by helping them focus on something other than what is distressing them at the moment. They are trying to solve their immediate problem, i.e., to reduce their emotional pain, and while that makes sense, the DBT therapist will point out to them, "Your short-term solution to pain brings with it even greater long-term suffering." Suicide, on the other hand, has as its purpose the permanent end to that person's suffering. However, even if people engage in parasuicidal behavior, they might accidentally cause enough damage to be lethal, or at some point make the decision to die by suicide. The moral of the story is that the underlying motivations for self-harm and suicide can be very different, but therapists and parents must take all incidents of self-injury very, very seriously.

Outcomes Studies

Research has demonstrated that DBT is effective for parasuicidal patients with BPD, patients with BPD and co-occurring substance use disorders, patients with eating disorders, and elderly patients with depression and personality disorders (Chapman, 2006). A 2020 study shows that patients who received DBT had significantly fewer suicide attempts, incidents of self-injury, and number of days hospitalized, compared with patients who received treatment as usual (Tebbett-Mock et al., 2020). Evidence also suggests that dialectical behavior therapy for adolescents (DBT-A), a modified version of DBT, is effective in treating adolescent self-harm, suicidality, and depression (Asarnow et al., 2021).

My Own Take on Using DBT with Children and Adolescents Who Self-Harm

DBT is now considered the gold standard for the treatment of patients who engage in self-harm or are chronically suicidal, and for good reason. Linehan and her colleagues have accumulated three decades' worth of research establishing its efficacy. However, as is the case with CBT, it simply doesn't help everyone. Virtually all of the children and adolescents we treat have already had extensive treatment using DBT, but they are still hurting themselves. In IFFT, we incorporate DBT into almost every individual and family therapy session, but far from just that alone. As a stand-alone treatment, there are many children and teens who do not benefit from DBT. Furthermore, DBT is difficult to implement in real-world practice. More on this in the final chapter of this book.

Combining DBT (and CBT) into a family-focused treatment plan is, in most cases, exactly the modification the child needs to really put self-harm behind them once and for all.

References

American Psychological Association. (2017, July). *What is cognitive behavioral therapy?* https://www.apa.org/ptsd-guideline/patients-and-families/cognitive-behavioral

Asarnow, J. R., Berk, M. S., Bedics, J., Adrian, M., Gallop, R., Cohen, J., Korslund, K., Hughes, J., Avina, C., Linehan, M. M., & McCauley, E. (2021). Dialectical behavior therapy for suicidal self-harming youth: Emotion regulation, mechanisms, and mediators. *Journal of the American Academy of Child and Adolescent Psychiatry*, 60(9), 1105–1115.e4. 10.1016/j.jaac.2021.01.016

Beck Institute. (n.d.-a). *The history of cognitive behavior therapy.* https://cares. beckinstitute.org/about-cbt/history-of-cbt/

Beck Institute. (n.d.-b). *Understanding CBT.* https://beckinstitute.org/about/ understanding-cbt/

Behavioral Tech. (n.d.). *What is dialectical behavior therapy (DBT)?* https:// behavioraltech.org/resources/faqs/dialectical-behavior-therapy-dbt/

Bryan, C. J., Peterson, A. L., & Rudd, M. D. (2018). Differential effects of brief CBT versus treatment as usual on posttreatment suicide attempts among groups of suicidal patients. *Psychiatric Services, 69*(6), 703–709. 10.1176/ appi.ps.201700452

Burns, D. D. (1980). *Feeling good: The new mood therapy.* William Morrow and Company.

Chan, M. K. Y., Bhatti, H., Meader, N., Stockton, S., Evans, J., O'Connor, R. C., Kapur, N., & Kendall, T. (2016). Predicting suicide following self-harm: Systematic review of risk factors and risk scales. *The British Journal of Psychiatry, 209*(4), 277–283. 10.1192/bjp.bp.115.170050

Chapman, A. L. (2006). Dialectical behavior therapy: Current indications and unique elements. *Psychiatry, 3*(9), 62–68.

Gilbert, A. C., DeYoung, L. L. A., Barthelemy, C. M., Jenkins, G. A., MacPherson, H. A., Kim, K. L., Kudinova, A. Y., Radoeva, P. D., & Dickstein, D. P. (2020). The treatment of suicide and self-injurious behaviors in children and adolescents. *Current Treatment Options in Psychiatry, 7*, 39–52. 10.1007/s40501-020-00201-3

Kann, L., Kinchen, S., Shanklin, S. L., Flint, K. H., Hawkins, J., Harris, W. A., Lowry, R., Olsen, E. O., McManus, T., Chyen, D., Whittle, L., Taylor, E., Demissie, Z., Brener, N., Thornton, J., Moore, J., & Zaza, S. (2014). *Youth risk behavior surveillance—United States, 2013* (Morbidity and Mortality Weekly Report Surveillance Summaries, Volume 63, Number 4). U.S. Department of Health and Human Services, Centers for Disease Control and Prevention, Center for Surveillance, Epidemiology, and Laboratory Services. https://www.cdc.gov/ mmwr/pdf/ss/ss6304.pdf

Leuzinger-Bohleber, M., Hautzinger, M., Fiedler, G., Keller, W., Bahrke, U., Kallenbach, L., Kaufhold, J., Ernst, M., Negele, A., Schoett, M., Küchenhoff, H., Günther, F., Rüger, B., & Beutel, B. (2019). Outcome of psychoanalytic and cognitive-behavioural long-term therapy with chronically depressed patients: A controlled trial with preferential and randomized allocation. *The Canadian Journal of Psychiatry, 64*(1), 47–58. 10.1177/0706743718780340

Linehan, M. M., & Wilks, C. R. (2015). The course and evolution of dialectical behavior therapy. *American Journal of Psychotherapy, 69*(2), 97–110. 10.1176/ appi.psychotherapy.2015.69.2.97

Linehan, M. M., Armstrong, H. E., Suarez, A., Allmon, D., & Heard, H. L. (1991). Cognitive-behavioral treatment of chronically parasuicidal borderline patients. *Archives of General Psychiatry, 48*(12), 1060–1064. 10.1001/archpsyc.1991. 01810360024003

Muehlenkamp, J. J., Claes, L., Havertape, L., & Plener, P. L. (2012). International prevalence of adolescent non-suicidal self-injury and deliberate self-harm. *Child and Adolescent Psychiatry and Mental Health, 6*, Article 10. 10.1186/1753-2000-6-10

National Institute of Mental Health. (n.d.-a). *Borderline personality disorder*. U.S. Department of Health and Human Services, National Institutes of Health. https://www.nimh.nih.gov/health/topics/borderline-personality-disorder

National Institute of Mental Health. (n.d.-b). *Suicide*. U.S. Department of Health and Human Services, National Institutes of Health. Retrieved May 16, 2023, from https://www.nimh.nih.gov/health/statistics/suicide

Seligman, L. D., & Ollendick, T. H. (2011). Cognitive-behavioral therapy for anxiety disorders in youth. *Child and Adolescent Psychiatric Clinics of North America*, 20(2), 217–238. 10.1016/j.chc.2011.01.003

Stewart, J. G., Valeri, L., Esposito, E. C., & Auerbach, R. P. (2018). Peer victimization and suicidal thoughts and behaviors in depressed adolescents. *Journal of Abnormal Child Psychology*, 46(3), 581–596. 10.1007/s10802-017-0304-7

Tebbett-Mock, A. A., Saito, E., McGee, M., Woloszyn, P., & Venuti, M. (2020). Efficacy of dialectical behavior therapy versus treatment as usual for acute-care inpatient adolescents. *Journal of the American Academy of Child and Adolescent Psychiatry*, 59(1), 149–156. 10.1016/j.jaac.2019.01.020

Whitlock, J., Eckenrode, J., & Silverman, D. (2006). Self-injurious behaviors in a college population. *Pediatrics*, 117(6), 1939–1948. 10.1542/peds.2005-2543

Wootton, B. M., Bragdon, L. B., Steinman, S. A., & Tolin, D. F. (2015). Three-year outcomes of adults with anxiety and related disorders following cognitive-behavioral therapy in a non-research clinical setting. *Journal of Anxiety Disorders*, 31, 28–31. 10.1016/j.janxdis.2015.01.007

World Health Organization. (2021, June 17). *Suicide*. Retrieved May 16, 2023, from https://www.who.int/news-room/fact-sheets/detail/suicide

7 The Treatment of Suicide and Self-Harm from a Family-Focused Perspective

We will turn our attention now to treatment itself, from a family-focused perspective. The effective treatment of suicidal and self-harming behaviors undoubtedly incorporates elements of CBT and DBT, but there is quite a bit more to it, as we shall see. The various clinical interventions, techniques, and strategies discussed in this chapter constitute a treatment package, with each element serving an important function.

As is the case with DBT, treating self-harm and suicidal urges begins with the premise that keeping the child safe is the primary focus at the start of treatment. Keeping the child alive is obviously the critical goal, and to paraphrase what Linehan somewhat bluntly and irreverently says to her patients, "You realize if you were dead, therapy is not going to work?" (Wick, 2005). These are the behaviors that brought the child and family into treatment in the first place, and addressing safety should always be at the top of any treatment hierarchy.

While there can be numerous other treatment issues to address, such as improved communication, reducing heat and reactivity in a family, improving the family's ability to solve problems peacefully and collaboratively, disrupting the influences of a negative peer group or social media, and so on, safety is of the utmost importance. Although there is a focus on reducing or eliminating self-harm in every session, this doesn't mean that in IFFT we wait to address other important issues or family dynamics. Quite the contrary. Self-harm and suicidal urges are fueled by a number of environmental and situational influences, as we have discussed; thus, in IFFT these are topics that are addressed from the very first session onward. In a nutshell, treatment is focused on any potential issues that are problematic, and not limited to self-harming urges and behaviors.

Distinguishing Depression from Anger and Why It Matters

In Chapter 1, we discussed the current thinking on some of the likely contributors to the increased prevalence of suicide and self-harm among

DOI: 10.4324/9781003397366-10

children and adolescents. When looking for underlying causes, depression is most often identified. Certainly, children who are depressed have an increased likelihood of hurting themselves, and developing an effective treatment plan designed to alleviate depressed mood is essential.

However, as is often the case, I believe when adults try to understand or account for a child's behavior, we have a tendency to arrive at causal explanations that would make sense to us if we were to hurt ourselves. Most of us believe that another adult would take their life only if they had become extremely depressed and hopeless, such that taking their life seemed like the only way to end their suffering. While perhaps often true with adults (and obviously sometimes with children and teens as well), I think it is a mistake to see young people through this same adult explanatory lens.

I have learned that children and teens think very, very differently from adults. This is likely due to the fact that their brains have yet to fully mature, and their capacity for abstract thought has not yet fully developed. They think much more concretely than adults, often in black-and-white terms (one of the ten cognitive distortions), and if you combine this with a significant lack of life experience, maturity, and wisdom, their views can be very difficult to understand when seen from an adult brain's perspective. I believe this often leads us to the wrong conclusion about what underlies their motivations and behavior. Think of it as a kind of cultural difference—you have to get inside their young heads to really understand how they see things, especially when it comes to something as serious as self-harm and suicide.

In my clinical experience, I do not find that depression is the leading contributor to self-harm urges. There are driving forces that are often overlooked in a discussion of self-harm among children and teens that are far more prevalent and significant: Anger and a desire for significance.

Let's begin with anger. I spend an awful lot of time worried about my patients. These are children and adolescents with serious mental health challenges, many of whom have hurt themselves many times, attempted to take their lives, or both and probably will again. But in truth, and I know this sounds a bit counterintuitive, I don't worry as much about my patients who are depressed. We know they are depressed, we can see it—their mood is obviously low because they tell us, and their behavior is consistent with someone who is depressed (lethargic, unhappy, and often very inactive). This usually makes their distress obvious and top of mind (ours and their parents), making it far more likely that collectively we will all lean in and offer immediate support.

The kids I worry about the most, the ones that always keep me up at night, are the ones who are angry and impulsive. Angry at their parents, angry at their peers, or just plain angry at the entire world. Something will happen to them—maybe it's being told no to a request, getting a consequence from their parents, experiencing a slight (or perceived slight) on social media (very common), and *just like that*, they impulsively cut themselves or swallow enough pills to end their life. In fact, one study found that almost half of people who had attempted suicide reported that the period between making the decision to do so and the actual suicide attempt was ten minutes or less (Deisenhammer et al., 2009). *Ten minutes.* That's the scariest part about it—it happens so quickly that there is often no opportunity for anyone to stop it.

There is often an "I'll show you" element in this type of self-harm. It's not revenge per se, more of a "Look what you did to me" type of thing, or "I'm really angry and now you're going to feel bad too." Kids have so little power in the world, not over their parents and not over their peers, and self-harm is in its own way a statement: *Enough*.

And there is another element to all of this. Arie Kruglanski, a professor of psychology at the University of Maryland, talks about what he calls a "quest for significance" as a driving force among mass shootings committed by those who are angry and disenfranchised. It is a way to get back at the world, to show that they matter. The driving force is triggered by experiencing a significant loss through humiliation and failure, resulting in a desire to regain significance and respect (Kruglanski, 2022).

This seems to me entirely consistent with what I know about how kids think. They do not consider the larger implications of things; for example, the fact that suicide is a permanent solution to a short-term problem, or that they would be cutting their life short over an event that 10 years from now they'd likely not even remember. In my experience with kids, they think things through exactly one inch into the future, and that's about all.

So yes, I do worry the most about angry and impulsive kids. From a treatment perspective, how one intervenes with a child who is depressed is going to look very different from working with a child who is impulsive and angry. With the latter, while DBT is useful in terms of improving emotion regulation and distress tolerance, a larger focus on CBT is likely more helpful to assist the patient with identifying distorted, negative thoughts that lead to anger, which ultimately drives the impulsive, self-destructive act.

Monitoring Phones and Other Devices to Increase Safety

A child or teen's phone is their conduit to the world, and my colleagues and I have found that it is common for kids to let their peers know about their thoughts or urges to hurt themselves well before their parents are aware of it. Sometimes this is done directly ("I just cut"), while at other times it's a more oblique reference ("I can't take this anymore and I'm just done.") In some cases, this results in a peer notifying their own parents who then contact our patient's parents, and in other cases the peer contacts our patient's parents directly. But in many, many instances, parents are in the dark and never learn that their child has told someone about hurting themselves. We highly recommend that parents with a suicidal or self-harming child electronically monitor their phones and other devices in order to give themselves an opportunity to immediately intervene. Several options exist for this, but we routinely recommend that parents use an application called Bark. Bark does not allow parents to read every message their child sends or receives, so it still allows some measure of privacy. It will, however, identify key words that are potentially worrisome, such as cut, suicide, pills, dead, and so on. Bark then sends the parent's phone an alert with sections of the message that contain this type of content.

Obtaining a Commitment to Reduce or Ideally Eliminate Self-Harm as a Primary Treatment Objective

Similar to DBT, treatment always starts with a focus on commitment to reducing self-harm. No treatment, no matter its potential to be helpful, is going to be of much value to a person who doesn't want it or doesn't see any reason to change. In the very first session, the IFFT clinician starts by asking the child what their level of commitment is to reducing or, ideally, eliminating self-harm (and psychiatric hospitalization if relevant, as we shall see in just a bit). There is empirical evidence that shows that when a commitment is made publicly, spoken out loud, or otherwise made explicit, it is much more likely that the commitment will be honored than when the commitment is left unspoken (Cialdini, 2001). For example, people who tell their friends and family that they are starting a new diet have a higher probability of sticking to the diet than people who decide to do it but do not tell anyone.

The conversation in the child's first individual therapy session relative to obtaining a public commitment flows like this:

Therapist (T):   So, if I can ask, your parents have told me that you sometimes hurt yourself. Is that true?

Child (C):   Yeah. Sometimes.

T: The kids I've worked with have told me different reasons why they do it. Usually what I hear is that cutting takes their mind off something else that's bothering them so it helps them feel better. Or that it just makes them feel better somehow. I don't want to put words in your mouth, but is there some of that going on for you maybe?

C: Maybe, I guess.

T: So if that's true for you, I'm guessing you probably don't think about hurting yourself when you're doing okay, things are great, and your mood is good, is that true?

C: Yeah, only when I'm sad or depressed.

T: Well, that makes sense then. You've got this thing you know how to do when you're sad or upset. And if it makes you feel better I can understand why you'd keep doing it. If I could show you a way to feel better faster without hurting yourself, would you be interested?

C: Maybe, yeah, I'd be interested.

[I've never once, not once, had anyone answer that question with a "no."]

T: Nice. Can I ask you this? On a scale of 1–10, how interested or committed are you in working on this, maybe even not hurting yourself at all, if I could teach you how to feel better faster and still stay safe? 10 being, yeah, I'm super committed, 1 being I'm not committed at all?

C: I don't know. A 5 maybe?

T: That's awesome. How come not a 10?

C: Because I'm not sure you can help so I'm not sure if I want to stop yet.

T: That's fair. And we really don't know each other yet do we, so being a little skeptical makes sense. Out of curiosity, though, how come it's not a 1?

C: Well, because my parents want me to stop. And I've got all these scars I don't like. And sometimes I end up in a psych hospital, which I really don't like.

T: Oh there's that too, yeah. The hospital, I forgot. Your stays in the hospital—those have been super helpful, right? Got a lot out of it?

[Side Note: I phrase it like this on purpose because I already know that's not true. I can use the child's disliking of the hospital to get a commitment on that, too. In IFFT, we work very hard to keep kids out of psychiatric hospitals unless it's absolutely necessary. I do not feel that any semblance of a normal adolescent life includes trips to a psychiatric hospital.]

C: No, it didn't do anything. I hated being there.

T: So, what's your commitment to staying out of the hospital then?

C: That's at a 9.

T:	Ok, cool, I'm with you on that too. Let me write that down before I forget: Hospital is a hard no. Okay, so quite a bit in it for you to work on not hurting yourself. So, what do you think, deal, want to work on this together maybe, you and me?
C:	I'll try, yeah.
T:	Awesome.

A similar conversation would then take place in the first family session. For example, the therapist, with the child's permission, would tell the parents about this discussion, letting them know that their child has committed to working on self-harm and praising the child's decision and maturity in making this commitment even if the commitment is weak. The therapist might reinforce the child's decision to commit by saying something like, "I have to call you out on something that's pretty impressive to me. You just started therapy and already you're doing hard things. Are you always like this—ready to step into doing hard things? I love that about you and how much wisdom it shows. Mom and Dad, do you agree? It's pretty cool, right?"

In IFFT, we believe that one of the most important factors in reducing self-harm over the course of treatment is the regularity with which the subject itself becomes a part of the discussion in each individual and family therapy session. There is just something about this process that seems to work. It indirectly communicates to the child that getting past this is very important, and by bringing self-harm up in some fashion in each session, it's also made clear that it's the focus of the entire family and everyone is committed to helping the child find alternate ways to cope and manage stress. Self-harm thrives in secrecy and the dark; this is the exact opposite.

Let us turn our attention now to specific interventions used by both the therapist and parents to address self-harm.

How a Parent Can Best Respond during a Self-Harm Event

There is no training in life that prepares a parent for how to respond when their child or teen says, "I just cut myself." Seeing cuts on a child's body is such an upsetting experience that words do not come easily, and often what parents say in the moment can be less than helpful. In the weekly parent sessions, we discuss why their response to self-harm can often set the stage for how the self-harm event will unfold, both immediately after the event itself and over the next several hours. If we are also working to reduce or prevent psychiatric hospitalization, the parents' immediate response becomes even more critical. In IFFT, we coach parents on the importance of staying calm and matter-of-fact in the face of any behavioral challenge, but this is particularly important if the child hurts themselves. The child is already upset or angry, or they would not have hurt themselves in the first place. If a parent becomes distraught or escalates, it would almost certainly cause the child to become further dysregulated, increasing the probability of more self-harm.

Often in the absence of coaching, most parents make comments that are not helpful, such as, "Again? I thought you were done with that?"; "How much longer do we need to keep doing this?"; "Look what you're doing to your body" or "Therapy isn't working." Parents are often understandably desperate to know why their child keeps hurting themselves, so they often ask, "Why did you do that?" I've found that "why" questions for children and teens are very hard for them. In most cases, they really don't know why they did it, but when pressed for an answer they will come up with some kind of explanation, which often doesn't hang together very well, and is very dissatisfying to the parent ("You made me mad" or "No one at school gives a shit about me"). While perhaps true or partially true, this is really not an explanation in the parent's mind for behavior that seems so mystifying and self-destructive. Interestingly, I find most adults don't do well with "why" questions either; their answers just tend to be longer but only slightly more illuminating. In truth, I think most of us really have no idea why we do what we do, we just do it. "How" questions tend to work much better: "How did that happen?" The phrasing alone subtly pulls for an explanation that includes the sequence of events (a behavior chain in the language of DBT) that led up to the self-harm, thereby making sense of what led the person to ultimately decide to hurt themselves.

An ideal first response that tends to work well is a simple, matter-of-fact but somewhat concerned, "Oh no, I'm sorry to hear that happened. I know that's been something you've been working on." The flow of this conversation between the parent and child, therefore, is as follows:

Parent (P): Oh no, I'm sorry to hear that happened. That's been something you've been working on. Feel like talking about it?

Child (C): No. I don't know.

P: How did that happen, do you think? What was going on?

C: I just got upset.

P: I see. I know sometimes you hurt yourself when you're upset so that makes sense. Want to tell me what happened?

C: I was messaging Jade and she told me my boyfriend was sexting this other girl and asking for nudes.

P: Oh I see, I'm so sorry, that must have been really painful to hear. Want some advice or would you like me to just listen?

C: Just listen.

> *[I believe that in our efforts to help, parents (and sometimes therapists) rush in far too quickly to offer advice or solutions. There's nothing wrong with that per se, but I find advice or problem-solving often comes far too early in the exchange. People need to be first heard and understood, and you have to spend some time doing this very early in the conversation. If you lead with soothing ("Oh I see, I'm so sorry …") and then validation ("… that must have been really painful to hear"), it seems to create a sense of intimacy and empathy, necessary precursors to any discussion on what to do about the problem. And some people don't want solutions at all; they just want you to empathize and listen, so I always like explicitly asking for consent before moving on to giving advice ("I have some ideas as to what might be helpful. Would it be okay with you if I shared them?")*

Parent (P):   Ok, I'll just listen. Just know that I love you and everything's going to be okay. And then let's clean up those cuts and get them taken care of.

If the child in the above example wants to talk more about what happened that's okay— but it's good for parents to remember that there are some problems they cannot fix. In the case of the boyfriend sexting another girl, that's something the child is going to have to fix themselves. If you rush in and try to do something about it, that denies the child the opportunity to learn how to successfully navigate an upsetting experience, cultivate the communication and assertiveness skills needed when another person hurts them, and develop a sense of competence that only comes from doing hard things. Rushing to fix is done with good intentions, obviously, as no one wants to see their child in pain. Certainly, there are times in which a child legitimately needs help and advice, but it is far better to let them try to solve their own problems and only step in when they really do need your help.

The Clinical Team's Immediate Response to a Self-Harm Event

In IFFT, we ask that parents reach out to the clinical team anytime there is a self-harm event. Our response would take into consideration a number of variables before making a decision as to how to best respond to the self-harm. One of our important goals with any family is sustainability; that is, teaching families the skills needed to successfully navigate difficult events on their own without our assistance. As I mentioned earlier in the book, I believe good therapists work hard to make themselves obsolete; we want to get in, help to the best of our ability, and get out of a family's life as quickly as possible. We definitely want to know about the self-harm event, and use our knowledge and understanding of this particular child and family to guide our response based on the following:

- How long has the team been working with the family? We are much more directive with newer families ("Here's what we think you should do ...") than we are with families who are farther along in treatment ("How would you like to handle this?").
- Are the parents able to stay reasonably calm in a situation like this, or should our initial focus be to start by helping with de-escalation and getting everyone better regulated again?
- What is this child's history of self-harm? Is it predominantly nonlethal (superficial cutting for example) or have they sometimes hurt themselves more seriously? The latter would require a greater focus on safety, such as considering whether to hospitalize the child.
- What is the nature of the self-harm in this instance? If the child requires medical care, we would make sure the parents take them to the ER.
- How motivated is this child to avoid hospitalization? The more motivated they are, the more we would help advocate on their behalf with the ER staff to safely return the child back home rather than send them to a hospital. If the child is motivated to stay out of the hospital, we capitalize on this and engage them in committing to safety and creating a safety plan, and help them advocate on their own behalf with the hospital clinician. Conversely, if the team feels hospitalization is warranted, we would do the reverse, i.e., work with the hospital clinician and advocate for the child's admission.
- What is the child's knowledge of and willingness to use DBT skills? An out-and-out rejection of the use of these skills ("The skills are stupid and don't work") tips us back in the direction of hospitalization because that indirectly speaks to the child's lack of commitment to staying safe.
- How well is this child connected to the individual therapist on our team? In newer cases, the child will not be as well-connected as in a more established case. In IFFT, children and teens are routinely given their therapist's cell numbers and are encouraged to reach out if they ever need help or coaching. Is this child likely to reach out if they feel they need to, or would they resist efforts by the therapist to directly speak with them?
- What is our overall assessment of safety? Previous patterns of self-harm and the answers to the questions above will guide whether we then conduct a more formal safety assessment by phone, which would involve a conversation directly with the child.

As the reader can see, these issues can be complex, and the various decision trees available require a great deal of thoughtfulness and skill. I tend to look at it like it's a math problem—multiple variables must be considered and manipulated simultaneously to, hopefully, arrive at the safest and most helpful solution, but a mistake is serious and possibly even deadly.

Let us take a brief detour for a moment and consider the role psychiatric hospitalization plays in all of this, and then we will return to this self-harm event and learn more about how the child's clinical team responds.

Psychiatric Hospitalization

Not all children and adolescents who hurt themselves require treatment in one of the approximately 1,800 psychiatric hospitals across the United States, although many of them do. When a child tries to take their life or hurt themselves (parasuicidal behavior), safety, obviously, becomes the primary concern. Often after a self-harm attempt, no one, neither the parent nor the treating therapist, can be certain whether the child might hurt themselves again. Having a safe environment available to closely monitor the child, review the medications they are on with a fresh set of eyes, and provide some immediate therapeutic support, can in many instances be a life-saving intervention. However, as an intervention, psychiatric hospitalization comes with some distinct, unanticipated consequences, and the potential for actual harm.

In my clinical experience, most parents who take their child to the emergency room for the first time have little to no understanding of the process that is about to unfold, and what little control they will actually have over it. I will describe this process in some detail to better inform parents who might someday be faced with hospitalization, in the hope of reducing some of the fears and concerns that can come along with this very serious intervention.

The ER is generally the first point of contact after a serious self-harm event. If the child or teen has ingested pills, they obviously require immediate medical care. Similarly, if there has been some type of self-harm event, for example, cutting that is beyond superficial, the child will also require medical attention. Parents are generally allowed to sit with their child in the ER, although not always, particularly if the child is escalated and angry with the parent for having taken them there (not an uncommon situation). The first task of the hospital is to medically stabilize the child, treat and suture wounds if necessary, and so forth.

It is important for parents to know that, at least for hospitals in the U.S., once you arrive at the ER due to self-harm, you cannot leave with your child even after they've been medically cleared. The child must be seen by a mental health staff person, usually a Master's level clinician (a licensed clinical social worker, marriage and family therapist, or the equivalent), to evaluate them and make the determination as to whether the child is safe to be released back to the parents and allowed to go home. The first contact with the hospital clinician is typically not quick; emergency rooms are often the most impacted and chaotic part of the hospital, with long wait times. Children and families are often required to remain in the ER for several hours before this person appears, virtually guaranteeing that any trip to the ER will often go late into the night or into the next morning. I suspect that a self-harming adolescent is a low priority for ER staff. I have sat with kids many, many times in the ER, and no one seems like they're in any particular hurry to get them out the door.

The decision to release the child back to their parents or place them on a 72-hour hold (a "5150," which refers to a section of the Welfare and Institutions Code) is made solely at the discretion of that clinician. This can be shocking to parents—that once in the ER, they lose the right to determine if their child comes back home with them, or is instead placed on a hold. Not only is this process generally unknown to parents, but the medical and mental health care systems do a poor job of educating families in advance about what to expect after they arrive at the ER. Often the child's treating therapist will simply tell parents, "Take them to the ER," without giving them an idea as to what lies in store for them. By law, a 5150 hold can be placed if the child is determined to be a danger to themselves (suicide attempt, suicidal thoughts, and self-harm), a danger to others (which is rare in my experience), or what's called "gravely disabled," which means that without hospitalization, the child would be unable to meet their own basic needs for food, clothing, and shelter (even rarer still, because children have families, so this is more often the case with adults).

The decision whether to psychiatrically hospitalize a child is based on an assessment of their safety at the present moment. Sometimes this is very clear-cut; for example, if the child says, "I'm not feeling safe and if I go home I'll probably hurt myself again." Sometimes, children and teens are not this clear and direct, and more often the clinical picture is a lot murkier. The conversation might go something like this:

Hospital Clinician (HC):	How are you feeling now? Your parents told me that you tried to take a bunch of Tylenol.
Child (C):	That's not true, they're lying.
HC:	Your lab work shows you took Tylenol.
C:	I never said I didn't take it, I said I didn't take a lot. I had a headache. That's what it's for, isn't it?

HC:	I think their worry is that maybe you were trying to hurt yourself. What do you think about that?
C:	I don't care what they think.
HC:	Well, my job is to figure out whether it's okay to send you home or have you go to a psychiatric hospital where you can be safe.
C:	I'm not going to a psych hospital.
HC:	Then I need to know if you're safe. If you go back home can you commit to being safe?
C:	I already told you that I didn't try to hurt myself.

Obviously, you can see why this exchange leaves the hospital clinician (and the parents) in the dark. In truth, the child often really has no idea if they're safe or not; they just know they don't want to be in the ER (usually they don't, but some kids do). Furthermore, if it's their first time in the ER, they're completely in the dark as to what is about to happen to them next, based on their responses to these questions. The clinician is likely going to decide to hospitalize this particular child based on their lack of commitment to safety and not taking accountability for what happened. If, instead, the child's last statement was, "Okay, so I was mad at my parents, but I just wanted to show them how mad I was. I was never going to kill myself and I'm not mad anymore, so I want to go home," the clinician would most likely develop some sort of safety plan with the parents (which basically means keeping a close eye on the child, getting an appointment soon with their therapist, etc.) and send the child home. Once the decision has been made to psychiatrically hospitalize the child, again, there is nothing the parents can do to prevent it. Also of note, the hospital often will not contact the child's existing therapist or psychiatrist to gather additional information that could be helpful in their assessment, making the process that much more frustrating to parents.

Beginning with the first point of contact in the ER, knowing that the hospital clinician is unlikely to contact us, the IFFT team makes a point of reaching out to them before they've made a final decision about hospitalization if possible. The importance of this contact cannot be overstated, as we often have vital information that will help them evaluate the child's current level of safety. Sometimes the hospital clinician is leaning toward hospitalizing the child when we feel they can return home safely, and, conversely, sometimes they are leaning away from hospitalization when we have information that the child is unsafe and that sending them home would be unwise.

It is very important for the reader to understand that not every self-harm event requires a trip to the ER and certainly not a stay in a psychiatric hospital (with the exception of an overdose attempt, due to its potential lethality). With a solid clinical plan and support in place, in many instances, a child can be stabilized at home and hospitalization can be avoided altogether. I worked with a family whose 15-year-old daughter had seven previous hospitalizations before starting IFFT. I asked the parents why this was the case, and they said, "That's what we were told to do. Take her to the ER so she can get the help she needs." You can see the obvious problem with this—the hospitalizations were completely avoidable had the right supports been in place. As it turned out, this girl's final hospitalization was in the week prior to starting IFFT.

If the decision is made to hospitalize, the hospital clinician will begin the challenging task of looking for a psychiatric hospital willing to take the child ("find a bed"). The U.S. is currently experiencing an urgent and worsening shortage of psychiatric beds (McBain et al., 2022). Competition for an available bed can be fierce, making it not uncommon for children and teens to be stuck in the ER for days or even weeks, awaiting a bed. Since hospitals have many more referrals than available beds, they can afford to be choosy, and choosy they are: If the child has a reputation, from previous stays at the hospital, of being disruptive on the unit, or a repeated pattern of going in and out of the hospital (derogatorily referred to as "frequent flyers"), the referral will be declined. The hospital staff will start by looking for a bed in the immediate geographical area, but since there are so few beds and referrals are often declined, parents generally have zero input as to how far away the child is ultimately placed. It is a miserable experience for the family to be parked in the ER for what feels like an eternity. Again, the process is generally not well explained to parents, who are learning as they go at a time when they are scared, confused, and badly sleep-deprived. On some occasions, after several days of searching for a bed without success, the child is so sick of being in the ER that they'll promise anything to get out (and the staff is sick of having them there too, honestly), so the hold is removed and the child goes home regardless of their actual current mental state.

The typical length of stay in a psychiatric hospital is generally between three days (this would be unusual) and several weeks, with about seven to ten days being the most common, in my experience. Days in the hospital are usually spent moving from one type of group therapy to another, for example, a DBT skills training group, the importance of sleep and self-care, and so on. Most of the children and adolescents that I have worked with have generally already had a healthy dose of all of this material, so they goof off or get into trouble with the other equally bored and not-so-stable patients.

The mission of the psychiatric hospital is short-term safety, and really not much else. It is not to achieve some lasting psychological change per se, and no one has the expectation that the child will be fundamentally changed as a result of their stay in the hospital. When they return home, they are generally more or less exactly the same person they were before going. The child will also come into contact with the hospital psychiatrist, who will likely adjust their current medication. In almost every case of hospitalization I've seen, the child's medication was changed in some way, most often increasing or decreasing the dose of an existing medication, adding a new medication, or both. It is rare for the hospital staff to collaborate with the child's existing outpatient psychiatrist, something that also can be frustrating for parents.

The Potential Harm of Hospitalization

As mentioned previously, psychiatric hospitalization can be highly valuable as an intervention when a child or adolescent is unsafe, but there are several potential unwanted consequences that can result from a stay in the hospital.

First, the experience overall, as one might imagine, can be very scary and upsetting, especially for younger children. A particularly egregious example of a young child needlessly hospitalized is that of a six-year-old girl in Florida who was placed on a 5150 hold by law enforcement (unknown to her parents) for being "out of control" at her school. Children are often terrified by the experience of being separated from their parents and placed into a loud, chaotic environment that brings them into contact with other children or teens, many of whom have far more serious problems. In addition to being a witness to some pretty scary stuff, there is an element of social contagion on the unit, i.e., children picking up on and imitating behaviors exhibited by other patients, thereby adopting new problematic behaviors not previously known to the child (Richardson et al., 2012). I am not judging the child in any way on this. As I've stated earlier in the book, kids just imitate each other. Negative peer influences on the unit are extremely powerful, resulting in all sorts of new challenges for the staff, the patients, and their parents. Furthermore, despite the hospital generally having rules that prohibit patients from exchanging contact information, they do so anyway. When a child returns home, they may remain in contact with other patients (often secretly) who themselves are struggling, thereby mutually reinforcing each other's problematic behavior.

While many children placed for the first time in a psychiatric hospital are so upset by the experience that they become highly motivated never to return, hospitalization can also have quite the opposite effect. Some children are drawn to the experience, either for a sense of community with peers, attention from the staff, escaping temporarily from a high-conflict home environment, or sometimes all of the above. In this situation, hospitalization can be so appealing that it actually reinforces the very behavior we are attempting to change ("If I cut myself, I know I'll get to go the hospital"), setting the stage for a pattern of repetitive hospitalization, sometimes as many as a dozen times in the space of a year.

In IFFT, as I stated previously, we begin with the premise that hospitalization ideally should not play any part in a typical child's life experience, nor is the need for it a particularly adaptive or helpful response to life challenges. We do advocate for hospitalization if a child or teen is unable to make a reasonable commitment to safety, but we work very, very hard to obtain this commitment. We make our position on this explicit to the parents at the onset of treatment ("We want to keep your child out of the hospital and develop alternatives that you and they can use that work better"). This is never a difficult sell to parents—who wants their kid to go to the hospital? (Never mind the crazy, marathon ordeals in the ER.) With the child themselves (similar to asking for a commitment to reduce or ideally eliminate self-harm), in the first session for a child who has a history of hospitalization, we ask for a commitment from them to work on not going back. For a child who did not like their experience in the hospital, this is a fairly easy commitment to obtain. From there, everyone— the parents, the clinical team, and the child—is working in unison toward this easily agreed-upon and very important goal.

For a child who has developed a reinforcement pattern of repeated hospitalizations, we also start by asking for the same commitment. In most cases, we can still obtain one fairly easily because, despite whatever draws them back to the hospital, most children, especially teens, recognize that the life they are currently living has gotten very far off track from that of their peers. (Or, as one kid put it, "I should be going to prom, not to the hospital.") They generally make the commitment to at least try to avoid the hospital—which I believe is sincere—but the problem, of course, is that their ability to successfully navigate their next upset can be so limited that their commitment not to get hospitalized vanishes in that moment. However, we are gently relentless in our pursuit to disrupt this pattern. We do so by disrupting self-harm in general because, as one might expect, if self-harm can be reduced there is inevitably a concurrent reduction in the frequency of hospitalizations. We also attempt to identify what it is about the hospital that is reinforcing for the child (for example, a sense of belonging to a peer group or wanting more adult empathy and attention) and look for ways to satisfy this need outside of the hospital.

Let us turn our attention now to the various clinical interventions that can be used to treat self-harm and suicidality effectively. I will describe the various clinical interventions that I believe are most effective and pull back the curtain on therapy for parents to see exactly what a therapist can do in a session to help the child.

Session Content and Clinical Objectives

Individual Therapy Sessions

By this time, the therapist has asked for a commitment to work on self-harm and begun to establish a good working relationship with the child or adolescent. What I find works best with most kids is to adopt a very relaxed, often playful demeanor. I am not a stiff therapist by any stretch of the imagination. I try to be as genuine and relatable as I can be, both with the child and their parents. Everyone has their own unique sense of humor, and I like to find it with my patients and use it as often as I can in session. I find if I can get someone to laugh in session, even for a moment, it's medicinal; it's hard to laugh and be miserable at the same time.

In IFFT, we ask parents to complete a daily log that is shared with and read by the treatment team. Parents are to create an entry each day that includes a few sentences about anything that went well during the week and anything that did not, so that when a child or parent comes into session, the therapist already has a good idea of the prior week and what needs clinical attention. Certainly, any self-harm event is going to need some unpacking. We find this daily log to be an extremely helpful tool in our work.

But with a child or teen, we would never start the session off with the unpacking. The therapist would want to spend some amount of time making small talk, getting a feel for the child's frame of mind, and warming them up a bit. The therapist's initial questions or comments relative to self-harm will be based on their read on the kid. If they can tell the child is off, they will spend much more time warming them up because we know going too quickly to some noteworthy event might cause them to shut down. If I know, for example, that the child had attended some event that I was sure went well, I'd spend a fair amount of time talking about it, again using my voice, tone, pace, facial expressions, and humor with the goal of warming them up enough to eventually get to the self-harm event itself.

In IFFT, we use reinforcement (praise and positive regard) liberally, sprinkled like water throughout every session. For example, if a child is managing to stick with a difficult topic the therapist might say, "I'm noticing something very cool that you're doing right now. We've been talking about something that's really hard for you and here you are pretty much hanging with the conversation from start to finish. That's kind of an adult thing to do. In fact, I know a lot of adults who wouldn't handle it as well as you did. I'm impressed." Children and teens with very serious mental health issues often feel like they get it wrong so much of the time, and almost always appreciate it when someone notices when they get it right (which is far more often than they're given credit for, I think). So every session starts with a focus on positives during the prior week, as many as the therapist can find, which sets the tone for what follows in the session and warms the child up so they're ready for the harder stuff.

At some point, when the timing feels right, the therapist will introduce the topic of self-harm ("Hey, your dad told me things were hard for you the other night, do you mind if we talk a little about that?"). Assuming the therapist gets some version of "yes" to that question, they will now embark on a mission with multiple goals in mind. The first goal, probably the most basic, is to hold the child in the space of the conversation. I find that most kids new to treatment are very unaccustomed to talking about hurting themselves. Presumably, it makes them feel uncomfortable and they don't see much value in it ("Why would I want to talk about that? When I think about it, I feel like shit, so it's better not to."). They are reticent with their parents as well and give them an "I don't know" or "I don't want to talk about it" when asked. This further distresses their parents, because they have no idea what is going through their child's mind, and the uncertainty is very scary for them.

Increasing a child's capacity to engage in difficult conversations in therapy is a must because if they can't (or won't), the therapist has only a limited ability to help. We have to be able to see the world from their perspective, understand the sequence of events as they saw or understood them, and hear the thoughts and beliefs (often with cognitive distortions) that culminated in the self-harm itself. Kids hurt themselves when they are distressed or angry, not when they are in a good mood. Therefore, I want to know what was distressing to them and why, as ultimately the goal is to teach the child better ways to navigate upsetting events so they can resist the urge to hurt themselves, or, even better still, have low or no urges to do so at all. Often, it's not an easy task to get a kid to open up in therapy; without the right skills to make this happen, sessions are going to stall out in a big way.

You can think of it as building up a muscle. We start slowly and through gradual, safe, and easy exposure to the process, the child gets more relaxed and better and better at it. They come to realize that it's not a bad experience to revisit a difficult event and that the therapist is there to lead the way using warmth, empathy, and support in abundance.

I find it's helpful, with kids who are highly avoidant about talking about hard things, to seek out entry points into the dialog, and only hold them gently in the conversation for the briefest of moments, sometimes well under a minute, and then exit that part of the conversation early and on purpose, before they beat me to it. If we've been talking about a negative event for a while and I get "I don't want to talk about this anymore," I know that I've gone on too long. If I suspect that's coming, I'll shift away from the topic and say something like, "Hey, that probably wasn't easy to talk about, but thank you. So what else is going on in your life?" My goal then would be to aim for a longer and longer discussion in each session, until I felt the child was comfortable enough to fully engage without shutting down. If the child likes you and trusts you, they'll eventually engage; they all do.

Okay, so now the child is talking. Where do we go from here?

In a word, *everywhere*.

I want to hear the story, as many details as I can get. What I find to be true, over and over again, is that when someone shares their perspective of an event, their thoughts, and their feelings, their behavior then starts to make an awful lot of sense. While I won't agree that the behavioral response, for example, cutting, is inevitable following some sequence of events, I can now see the world through their eyes and better understand how it played out the way it did. In the language of DBT, I would be conducting what is referred to as a behavior chain analysis, although I would never use that term with the child. It's too formal and sometimes both kids and adults find a chain analysis to be mildly annoying, so to begin a discussion by using the term would be starting us out on the wrong foot.

As we move through discussing the event, I'm looking for a number of different variables or opportunities that I can potentially use to my advantage. If done correctly, this discussion will offset the likelihood of a similar situation in the future culminating in self-harm. I'm looking for deflection points, opportunities to disrupt the flow of events, and things that I can suggest to the child that they might have done differently, thus resulting in a much better outcome. This might include skills or strategies that they could have used to lower their distress in the moment, making it more likely they would resist the urge to hurt themselves. For example, I might say "What do you think would have happened after your parents got mad at you if you had gone for a walk instead of going to your bedroom? Do you think you still would have hurt yourself?"

Consistent with CBT, I'm also listening for any potential distorted thinking and beliefs that led to whatever negative feelings the child experienced, typically resulting in anger, shame, frustration, sadness, disappointment, hopelessness, and so on. I do this because I know that a person's negative, distorted thoughts likely played a chief contributing role in the development of negative emotions. As I stated earlier in the chapter, negative thoughts plus negative emotions inform or drive behavior; in this case, the child hurts themselves rather than making a different, and safer, decision. I also want to be on the lookout for anything in the story that the child did right, no matter how small, so I can reinforce that behavior and potentially draw it out more often, with the goal of establishing it as a new behavioral habit. I will also try to validate their emotional experience liberally, as I know I cannot begin to help until the person feels heard and understood ("I can see why that situation was upsetting to you, it makes sense").

So, all in all, a pretty big agenda.

This is how all of this might flow in a session. In this example, I know from the parent log that a teen had a very bad experience at a birthday party, asked to be picked up early, and later that night cut in their bedroom.

Therapist (T):	So do you maybe want to talk about last night? Sounds like a hard night.
Child (C):	It wasn't good, that's for sure.
T:	Yeah, it seems like a bunch of different things happened all at once. Were you having kind of a rough day in general, or were things going good up until that point?
C:	No, my day was fine. Well, the morning anyway. Then I asked my mom to take me shopping and she said yes, so that was cool. But we were at the store and I wanted to buy something that she didn't want me to, and then she was a bitch. I told her she never lets me do anything, and then she yelled at me in the store and I yelled at her, so.
T:	I know this has come up between you and your mom before hasn't it? What you want to wear versus what she thinks is okay for you to wear?
C:	She never lets me wear what I want.
T:	So I'm guessing you picked out something that she didn't like?
C:	There was nothing wrong with it.
T:	You guys talked it out peacefully then? You each listened to the other, stayed chill, negotiated, and then finally agreed on something you could buy?
	[I asked it this way intentionally, knowing of course it didn't go like that. It's an easy, subtle way to point out that there was an alternative to how the situation was navigated that would have prevented the conflict.]
C:	Seriously? No. I got mad and she got mad.
T:	Oh. Then what happened?
C:	I went and sat in the car and she eventually came out and we left, but we didn't say anything to each other after that.

T: Is that when you started thinking about hurting yourself?

C: I thought about it but didn't.

T: Why not? You were mad.

C: I figured that was stupid so I just ignored her.

T: Hey, I know you don't like fighting with your mom and I'm really sorry that happened. But can I call you out in a good way on some things you did that I'm already seeing in this story that are pretty cool? Any idea what that might be?

C: That I didn't curse her out?

T: Yeah, I was thinking that too because I know there have been quite a few times where you were so mad at her that you did. And you got mad that day for sure, but it's pretty impressive that you mostly kept your cool. I also like the fact that you left the store without turning it into something bigger, and then made another good decision not to fight in the car and just go quiet. I love that your mom didn't try to engage you in the car because I'm guessing you were still pretty mad and needing space, and had she tried it probably wouldn't have gone so well. She probably knew that too. Oh, and the best part, you thought about hurting yourself but then didn't. Decided it would be stupid to do that, awesome. All very impressive and I love that you stayed safe and I'm sure your mom did too.

C: I guess, yeah.

        [I had assumed when this person began this story that it was going to be about the main event, what led up to the cutting. In my mind, I was conducting a chain analysis but as it turns out, not on the right thing. As the reader can see, this clearly is not the chain of events that directly precipitated the self-harm later in the evening, and by now I've figured this out. However, they did tell me the story, which means it was important to them in some way and I'm suspecting even though it wasn't a direct antecedent to self-harm, it likely put them in a negative mindset, probably increasing their vulnerability to something upsetting that occurred later in the day. But now we're here anyway, and I'm faced with a decision. The conflict with mom is worth spending some time on but I'm going to need to hurry up so I have time to get it. I take a subtle glance at the clock to see

how much time I have left in the session, do a quick calculation, and decide that I can probably linger here a bit and get some work done, and still have enough time to do a second chain on the cutting itself.]

T: That thought you had in the store, "My mom never lets me do anything." True do you think?

C: A little, yeah.

T: I didn't realize that about your mom. Seems like a pretty nice person to me, but maybe I misread her. So I'm thinking about a mom that never lets her kid do anything. Hmm. I'm guessing that mom would make them sleep in the closet underneath the stairs, probably treating her like the stepdaughter in Cinderella. Does she make you do a lot of mopping? She'd probably never let you leave the house, so many chores to do and all. But mice make really good friends, or so I hear.

[When I first challenge a negative thought I like to go big. I'll say it in a funny, exaggerated way because it almost always makes the person smile, and it's an easy way to point out (again, without directly pointing it out) that maybe the belief is a bit wonky. I would not do this with a new patient—not until they know me and I know them. This works when I'm tight with the kid and they're already accustomed to me saying funny things, but never in a disrespectful or unkind way. And I need to know this mom well—I'd never do this if a parent was actually mistreating this girl. It's a bit like what lawyers do in court—never ask a witness a question to which you don't already know the answer.]

C: Okay, very funny, I didn't say that! We don't even have stairs in our house.

T: Good thing. I find small spaces cozy myself. But let's get back to what happened. You were thinking that in the store right? She never lets you do anything. Maybe a little black-and-white thinking going on? Or discounting the positives—focusing on what she doesn't let you do versus the things she does, which we can make a list of if you like. *[I've already gone over with this kid the 10 cognitive distortions in prior sessions, so I can just call the distortions out by name here.]* If you believed that to be true, standing in the store, "My mom never lets me do anything," what feelings then trailed that thought?

C: I was pissed off.

T: Yep. And then I'm guessing because you were mad you started to push back. Argued with her. Then your mom pushed back too, and boom, now it's a fight.

C: That's pretty much it.

T: And if each of you were pushing back against the other, neither of you at that point is going to be in any kind of negotiating frame of mind. You can't negotiate and compromise on an outfit when everyone is mad and inflexible. Think your mom was out of line? The yelling part, yes, but not wanting you to wear something she didn't think was appropriate?

C: I think she's too strict.

T: On clothes, it sounds like she is strict more often than you'd prefer. But on everything? Isn't this the same mom who let you go to a concert last weekend?

C: Okay so she's not strict on everything.

        [At this point I could have spent more time gently challenging their negative thoughts, examining the evidence both for and against having a "strict" mom, and likely helping this person see that she is strict on some things, but certainly not everything. These are classic CBT moves by a therapist. I also would have given them some strategies on how to talk more effectively with their mom about clothing choices and how to better negotiate, or focus on acceptance if mom just isn't going to bend on this issue ("Sometimes parents do get to make the rules, that's just the truth of it."). But now I'm running out of time, and I want to quickly wrap this up and say something useful to close out this part of the conversation and move on to the main event.]

T: Look, you and your mom aren't always going to see it the same way and that's okay. And I get that it's frustrating for you, particularly since clothes have come up before. She's just doing the mom thing—looking out for you in her own way. And you're just doing the teenager thing—wanting some independence and say-so in your own life. There are no bad guys in this story. But I also know how much you both love each other and neither of you feels good after an argument. So you stayed safe, but this didn't put you in the best mood I'm guessing did it?

C: No.

T: What's the next part of this story?

C: I went to a birthday party at Makayla's house.

T: You mentioned last week that you were really looking forward to it.

C: I was. Until this other girl showed up that I didn't like. She talked shit about me on Instagram last year so I confronted her. She got super pissed and said I was fucking crazy because I had been in the hospital.

T: And then what?

C: She wasn't staying anyway so she eventually left the party.

T: Good that she left. But you weren't expecting any of that, were you? I bet you were really looking forward to this party but had no idea this girl was going to show up. Did it get any better after she left? I bet you were happy about that.

C: I was, but no it didn't get better. It got way worse. I didn't really know anyone there except Makayla and no one really talked to me much after that. I tried to stay positive but that's hard when basically everyone was ignoring me. And I thought Makayla should have stuck up for me, but she didn't. She kept acting like nothing happened. I sort of tried talking to Makayla's parents but they were busy with the party and kept telling me to go talk to the other girls. They didn't know what was going on. I went to the bathroom and cried but I don't think anyone noticed I was gone.

T: Hey, that must have been super painful. I know you love Makayla and you've been friends for a long time. And she was the only person you knew there. I can understand why you would be so hurt. That's a hard situation to be in, and I'd be hurt and sad too. How long did all that go on?

       [I can obviously see places where this kid made some decisions that weren't the best, like confronting someone at a party over some long-ago slight. I knew, though, that they were absolutely not ready for me to go there yet and had I tried, it would have been very poorly received. Better to slow down and hold them in that space, and just validate and use pace and the tone of my voice to soothe. That was easy for me because it really was an awful situation and I felt for them.]

C: I'm not sure how long. A few hours at least.

T: Really? You hung with that for a few hours? That's pretty impressive. And I know you—I bet you did your best to still interact with those girls.

C: I did. It wasn't working though.

T: You probably thought about calling your mom and asking her to come pick you up?

C: I was still pissed at her from earlier. But yeah, I did call her eventually.

T: What did she say about all that?

C: She was mad because she was out and now she had to come get me.

T: Oh. I bet that didn't make you feel any better, did it?

C: Fuck no. So I didn't talk to her in the car, and when we got home I went to my room and slammed the door. She knocked on the door but I told her to go away.

T: We're getting closer to the cutting part, aren't we?

C: Yeah. So my phone starts to blow up. Everyone at the party is messaging me and saying what a selfish bitch I was. I just needed to feel better, so I used a razor blade on my arm.

T: Can I see?

        [I don't know why I ask to see cuts on someone's arm, but I do every time. It's like a small moment of connection—them showing and me seeing something so personal. It's like I'm a witness to their suffering, or a metaphor for the cutting being truly out in the open now. It just feels right to do it.]

C: They're not too bad.

T: Remember earlier when I called you out on some of the really great ways you handled that thing with your mom in the store? Some parts of that story we worked on, but you did a lot of things right. What did you do right the night of the party?

C: Nothing. And I cut myself.

T: The cutting part isn't great, that's true, and I'm glad you're here so we can do some work on that. In fact, you've been doing really well with the self-harm lately—this is the first time in, what, months? But go with me on this—tell me the parts of that night you got right. If you get stuck I'll help.

C: Well, I confronted that stupid girl and as much as I wanted to hit her, I didn't.

T: I kinda get the temptation, but you were super smart not to hit her. Bet you wanted to bad, didn't you?

C: Yeah. And I also tried to stay at the party and talk to the girls, but that was way hard.

T: It was. But that took a lot of courage, and trying to make the best of something is a pretty grown-up response. That's it, those are the only good things, nothing else you can think of? You missed a bunch.

C: Like what?

T: Well, how about the fact that even though you were hurt and upset at the party you didn't tell those girls off? Or pull Makayla aside and let her have it. Again, bet you were tempted. Why didn't you?

C: Uh, that would have made it worse.

T: Very true. That would have blown things up for sure. I also liked that you tried talking to Makayla's parents, that was smart, but it didn't work well because they were busy with the party. How about the fact that you called your mom and got out of there? Not easy but you did. You were in the bathroom, but you stayed safe in there. Did you think about hurting yourself there?

C: Yeah. But I didn't.

T: Another smart move. You could have argued with your mom in the car, especially since she had kind of an attitude, but you didn't. You took space in your room, another good skill. But then you get there and all those shitty text messages started coming in. That was it, you were done—right?

C: Yeah. I know I shouldn't have cut myself. I'm pissed that I did it.

T: I'm kinda pissed at those not very nice girls who got so far into your head that you felt cutting was the only thing to do. But was it really? Let's look for places that day when you might have done something different that would have ended with you staying safe. Let's start with confronting that girl. I know you were pissed, but maybe not the thing to do? Or not there, anyway.

    [This feels like the right time to start looking at what this kid could have done differently. There's no way I could have done that earlier in the session.]

C: I could have just said nothing, or waited and messaged her the next day.

T: It's true. The party would have gone in a completely different way if you had. Or rather than "confronting" her the next day, maybe just try and talk it out? I find people usually don't do well with confrontations. And if you don't think she's worth the effort, maybe just not caring what this random, not very nice girl thinks? One of the cool things you'll find about getting older is that you stop caring as much about what other people think of you—your friends and family, yeah for sure, they matter—but the mean girls of the world? Not so much. What else might have worked after you got home?

C: I could have talked to my mom but we were mad at each other.

T: That's true. But what do you know about your mom? You think if she knew you were hurting so bad she wouldn't have cared and tried to help?

C: No, she would have cared and she would have talked to me, tried to make me feel better.

T: I know your mom pretty well and I think that's exactly what she would have done. And speaking of people who care and want to help, might there have been someone else you could have reached out to? Me for instance?

        [As is the case with DBT, both kids and their parents have access to their IFFT therapists outside of session after hours. This gives us the opportunity to intervene right away, often when we are needed the most. Gradually over the course of treatment, we reduce our accessibility to kids so they don't become too reliant on that, and encourage them to reach out to other supports, such as their parents and friends.]

C: I didn't text you because I knew you'd talk me out of cutting. At that point I was just so mad I didn't care, I just wanted to do it.

T: Mad or hurt?

C: Okay, hurt.

        [I often find feeling hurt underlies the emotion of feeling angry. It's really hard though for people to just sit with feeling hurt. When we feel angry, we feel righteous and powerful, which is much less painful.]

T: I'm guessing that you didn't think to maybe use any of your DBT skills?

        [This is one of the great contributions made by Marsha Linehan, the developer of DBT. In DBT, the idea is to

help patients build up a toolbox of skills, things they can do while dysregulated (upset) that will help them calm down, rather than resorting to self-harm as a way to feel better. In essence, the skills shift the person's focus from what is upsetting to them and buys enough time for their brain to eventually settle down and re-regulate itself. Emotions, including strong negative emotions, are like house guests; they come, stay for a while, but then eventually leave, you just have to wait long enough. Anytime self-harm occurs, it's really important to have a discussion about the use of skills, which in IFFT are taught in the weekly individual skills training sessions.]

C: I did, but I thought fuck those skills.

[Not an uncommon thing for kids (and adults) to say. Sometimes people just get to the point where they've had it with everything, and that's okay.]

T: If you had decided to use some skills, which ones might have helped?

C: A distract skill might have. I could have watched something on YouTube, or drawn maybe. Or use a self-soothe skill like taking a bath or making some hot chocolate.

T: Those might have worked, yes. Sounds like you're now re-committed to staying safe, is that right?

C: Yeah, for sure.

T: And in terms of me, what are you committing to that you'll do the next time you're hurt and upset like that?

C: I'll text you. And at least try to use my skills.

T: Awesome. And can I tell you what I admire about you, would that be okay?

C: I guess.

T: That you're able to come in here and trust me enough to talk about hard things. I know that's not easy, but I love how open and willing you are to talk through a difficult situation and allow me to walk you through it. I know a lot of kids your age who don't pull this off as beautifully as you. And how committed you are to doing the hard work and not hurting yourself. All pretty amazing stuff.

[The Makayla issue still needs work. First, because I know the relationship is really important to my patient and there might still be ways to salvage it. Second, because I know how easy it is for situations like these to bring a friendship to an end. The patient's thought "Makayla should have stuck up for me" is absolutely worth

examining. I can think of countless reasons why a teenager at her own birthday party might have handled the situation in a clumsy way; for example, not knowing what to do simply because it was awkward, not understanding how upset my patient was (probably because my patient worked hard not to let that show), thinking if she just pressed on with the party things would sort themselves out, and so on. None of these things make Makayla a bad friend, just a fairly normal, socially clumsy teenager. It would have been best to work on this in the same session, time permitting, so the two girls don't go a week without speaking, but this is the core of my patient's hurt (her interpretation of Makayla's behavior, or the story she's telling herself about it), and that discussion cannot be rushed.

On a side note, I know in advance of the session that this patient hurt themselves with a razor blade and I would want to get it. This is more of a symbolic gesture than a practical one, because in truth if someone is intent on harming themselves they can find a way to do it anytime and anywhere, and they know this just as well as I do. Plus, most people who engage in self-harm will frequently keep all kinds of sharp objects within easy access, but often hidden, so their parents can't find them. If I knew the patient had the razor in their possession, I would probably just ask for it right then but in a funny way, like "Okay you know what I'm about to say next right? Hand it over. Help your therapist not worry about you so he can sleep better tonight." I might get a little pushback but I find if I'm easy about it and go slowly, almost everyone hands over sharps. In fact, I have a drawer in my office full of them, and I tell people they can have them back as soon as they don't want them anymore. If the blade is at home, I'll ask the child to give it to their parents that day and text me so I know it's done, and then I'll text the parents just to make sure.]

Family Therapy Sessions

In IFFT, a self-harm event would be discussed and unpacked whenever possible in an individual therapy session prior to the family therapy session. The rationale for this is our observation that children and teens more readily open up and are able to talk through difficult subjects for the first time without their parents in the room, especially for new patients. Doing so also allows the therapist to collaborate with the child and agree on how much information is shared in the family therapy session. Like all therapists, an IFFT therapist does not share everything a child reveals in their individual sessions, but the therapist does talk about the big things in family therapy, and self-harm is a big thing. We feel it's important for parents to know about any self-harm, and we make that clear to kids at the start of treatment.

It's very rare for a self-harm episode to occur without the child telling one of us about it, likely because as mentioned previously, we work hard to establish a culture of openness and transparency around self-harm. It can also be very helpful to prepare a child in the individual session as to how they are going to speak to their parents in the family session about what occurred, in order for them to communicate effectively with them. And sometimes, if the parents don't already know about a self-harm episode, it can be unsettling for kids to tell them about it in session, and they often need quite a bit of help doing so.

The goal of the family therapy session is not to unpack the self-harm event at the same level of detail that occurred in the individual session. That is mostly a child-focused intervention, i.e., how the child could have handled that situation differently and any DBT skills they might have used to reduce the urge to self-harm, such that they could tolerate their distress and stay safe. Rather, in the family therapy session, the goal is to discuss and process the self-harm as it relates to the whole family. This can take several forms, but most commonly this falls into two categories: First, to what degree the self-harm is related to some sort of family issue, event, or dynamic, and second, to what degree, if any, the family might have been available to play some role in being a helpful buffer against the self-harm thus offsetting the event itself.

Self-Harm as It Relates to the Family

In many instances of self-harm, the child is reacting in a negative way to some sort of family conflict. In fact, in my experience, family conflict is often a precipitant to self-harm among children and teens, second only to conflict with peers. I believe this is why a family-focused approach is so vital, as it allows the clinician to effectively disrupt these dynamics and improve upon them, something an individual therapist is unable to do on their own. If conflict in the home is reduced, self-harm is also reduced in a corresponding manner.

Conflict in families related to self-harm can occur for a number of reasons. This can be a situation in which the child or adolescent wants something they can't have (being told no), a heated argument (which often results from being told no), breaking a rule of some sort (either being spoken to about that broken rule, and/or possibly receiving a consequence), a heated family argument (a gradual escalation of angry exchanges, likely the result of the principle mirroring and matching and a tug-of-war), or a response to some sort of perceived slight or critical comment from a family member (for example, a sibling might refer to the child as "the crazy one in the family").

These types of occurrences are often a launching point for strong negative emotions, which is an obvious vulnerability for self-harm. Typically, after a family conflict, most children will retreat to their bedroom in an angry or despondent frame of mind. Some will hurt themselves right away, while others will ruminate for a while and then ultimately make the decision to hurt themselves. A self-harm event can be a result of being depressed and hopeless, but as discussed previously, more often it is an angry, impulsive act. The goal of family therapy (and parent therapy) is to bring these negative family dynamics out into the open and identify alternatives so that positive change can occur.

Again, due to the daily log completed by parents, as well as any after-hours text or phone calls that occurred with the parents or the child with the IFFT team prior to the family therapy session, the therapist already knows what has happened and is ready to discuss the events in session. The therapist has also very likely already met for an individual session with the child, and now everyone is ready to get to work.

The family therapy session essentially mirrors the same basic sequence and flow of an individual session. The therapist will not jump to the conflict or self-harm right away and will instead warm up the child and family by identifying positives from the prior week. Focusing on positives also gives the therapist an opportunity to read the room and assess the emotional readiness of the child and family to begin a discussion about what occurred. When it's time to start, the therapist might begin by asking the parents, "So I know last night was hard for you guys. Can one of you start and fill me in on the details?" We often ask the parents to start off the discussion, because the therapist has already met with the child and they have a good understanding of how the child sees it.

An IFFT family therapist is very directive and highly active in the session. Families can, and often do, erupt at a moment's notice in the session, especially if they are all still angry or feeling misunderstood or mistreated in some way. The therapist must always disrupt negative or hostile exchanges that might unfold ("Wait, hold on, this is going too fast for me and I can't take it all in. Now Mom, can you tell me what you meant by ... ?"). And to the child, with their palm up, the therapist might say, "I know there's a lot you want to say and I promise I'll give you the chance in just a sec, I want to hear your dad out and then you can add what you'd like to share." This provides an opportunity to slow down the pace of the conversation, gather more information, model better and more effective communication, and truthfully, it gives the therapist time to think about their next move because it's hard to strategize when everyone is yelling. Typically, I will only allow two or three heated, argumentative back-and-forth exchanges between the parent and the child before stepping in and disrupting it. There's no value whatsoever in just letting people argue in session; that's exactly what they do at home and I'm there to teach them how to do it differently.

Family therapy is where the rubber meets the road in terms of communication: Listening to what the other person is saying (not just waiting for your turn to fire something back); giving others a chance to speak without interrupting them; staying well-regulated emotionally even if one person disagrees with the other; and approaching problems in a collaborative, loving way. These skills, had they been used on the day of the self-harm event, might have minimized the conflict and lowered reactivity, thereby reducing the probability of self-harm. The therapist is attempting a do-over of sorts: Talking in detail now about the past conflict but supporting the family to do so in a kinder way with a far better outcome.

The discussion at its core is also conducting a second family-based chain analysis. The therapist helps the family identify where, over the course of the day in question, other (better) decisions could have been made by calling out (nicely) behaviors that didn't work and examining alternative behaviors that would have been more effective. For example, "Telling your mom to fuck off is not a good opener to negotiating for something that you want, but staying respectful is," or to the parent, "I know it can be easy to get sucked into a heated back and forth, but it's best to disengage and walk away, and then circle back to the discussion after everyone has calmed down."

This is also the time and place to clarify any misunderstandings that likely arose during the conflict. It's surprising how often people overreact and make bad decisions in situations simply because they don't have all of the available information and fill in their information gaps with bad data. The family therapist will also be on the lookout for any cognitive distortions that lead a family member to misinterpret another person's motives or intentions. The final part of the discussion will be for family members to reach a new agreement, and formally (out loud) commit to it ("Okay from now on if I'm in that situation again here's what I'll do differently").

Self-Harm Not Related to Family

Children and teens can often hurt themselves as a response to a problem or situation completely unrelated to family, most commonly as I've stated due to a conflict with peers. Family still has the potential to offer the child comfort and support; however, they cannot do so if they are unaware of the situation or if the child is in pain or upset. Many children and teens who hurt themselves become isolated and disconnected from their families, the very people who are in the best position to help support them and perhaps even offer some decent advice. This is, in part, the rationale for talking about self-harm in every family therapy session, including situations in which the parents were not involved. We are helping to create a culture within the family in which seeking out one's parents becomes okay, normalized, and self-reinforcing (that is, the child gets a consistently positive and helpful response from their parents, making it more likely they'll seek them out in the future when it's helpful for them to do so).

If a child or teen is not routinely disclosing self-harm to parents, one of the goals in family therapy is to positively disrupt that dynamic by assessing what might be motivating the child to keep their parents in the dark. While there can be numerous incentives for the child not to disclose self-harm (shame, embarrassment, a conflict arising within a secret relationship with a peer, etc.), we want to make sure the parents' response to self-harm isn't a less-than-ideal one, which is why we coach parents on how best to respond when they learn of a self-harm event. We want to make it easy for kids to come to their parents and remove any barriers in their path to doing so.

Similarly, along the lines of a family as a buffer, in every family therapy session, we also focus on and heavily reinforce anytime a child experiences a difficult situation, either within or outside the family, and successfully manages to stay safe and not hurt themselves. Stressful events, somewhat counter-intuitively, can be a cause for great celebration. Parents, as always, are very powerful as reinforcers; therefore, calling a child out in a positive way in session is a very potent intervention ("That was a tough situation you were in and you handled it in a very mature way. It's impressive to me that you got through it, you handled it beautifully, and you stayed safe at the same time. I hope nothing like that happens to you again, but if it does I'm confident you'll get through it successfully then, too. If there is anything I could have said or done that would have been helpful, please let me know").

Parent Therapy

The important role that parents play in the treatment of self-harm and suicide cannot be overstated. As put succinctly by Guy Diamond, Gary Diamond, and Suzanne Levy, the developers of *Attachment-Based Family Therapy* (ABFT): "The quality of interpersonal relationships within families can precipitate, exacerbate, or buffer against childhood mental illness." (Diamond et al., 2014).

When I speak at a conference or a workshop I have, on occasion, tried to paraphrase and improve upon this sentence, but I finally gave up and just quote it directly because it's perfect just as it is. Parents are not necessarily the cause of their child's mental health condition (abusive parents being a clear exception), but even the most loving parents can inadvertently make things worse and miss out on opportunities to make things better. In a nutshell, the goal of parent therapy in the treatment of self-harm is for the therapist to identify and mitigate any potential behaviors of the parents that might be making their child's mental health symptoms worse and draw out and enhance those behaviors that can help a child better navigate stressful events or situations that might precipitate self-harm or suicidal thoughts.

There are numerous techniques and interventions used in IFFT parent therapy, relative to addressing self-harm. These include the importance of parents moving away from reactivity (raising their voice and being sometimes harsh rather than gentle), avoiding tug-of-war, not overly relying on consequences or other forms of discipline that are ineffective, avoiding unnecessary power struggles, and so on. All of these techniques (and many more) are taught to all parents receiving IFFT, with some covered in more detail than others, depending on the needs of the individual family. Some families already do a great job remaining matter-of-fact in the face of challenging behavior, so perhaps we would touch on that just briefly, and focus on other areas that might require some work.

Similar to individual and family sessions, parent sessions place an emphasis on processing a problematic event (again, a chain analysis) in order to identify various opportunities in which the parent might have done something differently. I believe that nearly all parents are well-intentioned and infinitely love their children, but they simply do not know what to do in the face of behavior that is scary and difficult to understand, especially self-harm. This seems quite understandable; no prior life experience is going to even remotely prepare a parent who is seeing cuts on their child's arm for the first time or learning that their child tried to intentionally overdose. Parents are hungry for knowledge and concrete advice that actually works ("What do I do when this happens?"), and they rely on the expertise and skill of the parent therapist to teach them what works and what does not. Raising your voice in anger at your kids does not work, falling into the trap of a back-and-forth argument does not work, and trying to change behavior through excessive reliance on consequences does not work; however, there are many, many alternatives that work beautifully.

The parents' role in helping their child reduce self-harm isn't an easy one by any stretch of the imagination. In Chapter 3 we discussed "righting the ship," that is, trying to return a sense of normalcy to a family that, in many ways, has gotten very far off course. In the case of a child who self-harms, this is the most challenging situation of all because often by the time a family presents for treatment, family life has ground to a veritable halt. The child has hurt themselves and, when this occurs, parents almost always try to reduce the child's stress in some way, most often by not asking much of them. Many of the normal expectations typically placed on a child are suspended, such as spending less time on devices, spending less time in their bedrooms and more with family, helping out around the house, doing homework, or even going to school at all. Therapists "fall into the pool" on this as well—many of the parents we work with have been told by previous therapists to "not stress" the child and to back off on limits and expectations. This usually translates into not asking anything of them and accepting all kinds of behavior that previously would have been unacceptable (disrespect for example, or no longer doing homework). This is fine as a short-term intervention (lowering stress), but if maintained over the long term, asking nothing of the child causes many issues that are increasingly problematic. To the best of my knowledge, the treatment for depression and self-harm is not spending more time in a dark bedroom, glued to a phone. It's the ongoing cycle of lowered expectations, increased isolation, withdrawal from healthy, age-typical activities, and less time with family, which must be disrupted and become the focus in the parent therapy sessions.

How is this done when a child threatens suicide if you ask them to spend less time on their phone, tells you that time on their phone is the only thing that's keeping them alive, or that without their phone they'd be even more depressed? These are all very common statements made by self-harming kids, and because parents are understandably afraid that the worst might happen, it becomes very easy for them to back down and stop asking things of the child or teen. The problem is that for most people, when little is asked of them, they give you exactly that, little. And while children and teens might appear somewhat content in this greatly diminished life, it doesn't change anything. They still cut and report feeling miserable.

Self-harm and depression can often serve a function. If a kid learns that when they hurt themselves, their parents then back off from age-typical expectations, the child then has an incentive to continue engaging in the self-harming behaviors. We see this again and again in our work. The best way to remove this incentive is for parents to resume asking kids to do hard things so that the function of the self-harming behaviors becomes neutralized. We will talk more about the functional aspects of childhood mental health conditions later in the book.

The only way to change this situation is to, well, change this situation. In parent sessions, we discuss the importance of getting the child or teen out of their bedroom and back into the world and help them re-engage with their family, a positive peer group, school, and siblings, and to contribute to the household in some meaningful way such as doing chores.

As one might expect, this temporarily stresses the child and the family system, and can briefly increase the risk of self-harm. However, in IFFT, this process is done very slowly and carefully, starting with small things, like showering each day or going for a walk. We are very careful to balance safety with change, and this strategy has been shown repeatedly to be an effective one.

In short, IFFT parent sessions are focused on reducing problematic family behaviors, especially those of the parents, that might be having a negative impact on the child's well-being, increasing the probability of self-harm. We identify and teach effective, alternative behaviors for managing challenging behaviors, and then embark on a journey to help the child resume a normal life as quickly as possible, one that does not include hurting themselves.

Skills Training

All children in IFFT have a second clinician they work with to learn and practice DBT skills in a 1:1 setting. DBT advocates for skills to be taught in a group setting; however, we find that doesn't work as well for adolescents, particularly if some members of the group are not as firmly committed to reducing self-harm as we would prefer. Additionally, a 1:1 setting is obviously much more personalized, and the clinician can draw from events of the prior week and target skills training directly to a recent event.

The Expected Course of Treatment

Self-harm in most instances is highly treatable. However as one might guess, it rarely disappears overnight, even if the child or teen is receiving effective treatment. As far as I can recall, I have only encountered a handful of cases in which an adolescent with a very significant history of self-harm and multiple hospitalizations started IFFT and never hurt themselves or were hospitalized from that moment on. It does happen, but much more commonly we find the self-harming behavior does not respond to treatment right away and the child will continue to hurt themselves at least for a while, sometimes as much as a few months into treatment. It takes time for us to unpack everything that is going on and implement the multitude of strategies described in this book. In most cases, the self-harm gradually begins to taper off, becoming less and less frequent. Conversely, as one might expect, we see a gradual increase in the child's ability to successfully navigate stressful situations while still staying safe. Self-harm is a complicated matter and it's not surprising that it takes a bit of time to figure out all of the various situational elements that are coming into play, and then effectively mitigating or disrupting each of them.

It is important for parents to be made aware of this at the outset of treatment, as it can be understandably disheartening if a child doesn't seem to be getting any better in the first few weeks. Additionally, some children and teens are able to stay safe for several months after self-harm has gradually tapered off, and then, for various reasons, the child will experience another self-harm event. In my experience, however, in the vast majority of cases, a self-harm event of this nature represents more of an outlier, a one-off so to speak, and generally does not result in a re-emergence of self-harm at the same frequency with which it was occurring at the start of treatment. This can throw parents off and be discouraging, so predicting this possibility in advance will go a long way to helping parents remain hopeful and optimistic, should it occur.

What Treatment Components Are Most Helpful?

In truth, I don't know which of the various strategies and techniques outlined in this chapter play the largest role in the effectiveness of the treatment. Other models of family therapy have attempted to parse out and test their various treatment components, and have produced some insights. For example, in one study on functional family therapy (FFT), the authors report that the ability of the therapist to quickly establish a "balanced alliance," i.e., not obviously siding too often with the parent or with the child, is essential for retaining the family in treatment (Robbins et al., 2003). I'll summarize here what I believe intuitively matters the most in IFFT relative to effectively treating suicide and self-harm, but I'll let the reader draw their own conclusions.

I believe there is something very important about the regularity of weekly sessions, and the fact that self-harm and/or suicidal urges are at least part of the focus in each session, either to unpack a self-harm event or to reinforce the absence of self-harm. This regularity keeps the focus on the self-harm and subtly communicates to the child that reducing it is of utmost importance.

I also believe that having the family speak openly and transparently about self-harm acclimates the child to talking about it easily with their parents, allowing the parents to lean in and offer much-needed support. As mentioned, in IFFT, we routinely incorporate CBT and DBT into nearly every session, which seems a clinical must, given their empirical support, but folding these treatments into a larger family-focused approach significantly enhances the effectiveness of both treatments to a far greater degree than when they are delivered in isolation. (Almost every child or adolescent we treat for serious self-harm has already received a healthy dose of both CBT and DBT, but has not improved until the family component was added.)

Additionally, I've yet to meet a single family of a self-harming child that was not inadvertently engaging in at least some behaviors that were making the child's problem worse or would not benefit from learning alternative, more supportive behaviors that help. Again, this is not in any way a judgment on the parent; rather it's an indication of how difficult it is to parent a self-harming child, and how essential it is to develop a better skill set. IFFT is a very directive treatment because parents absolutely want to know, concretely, what they can do differently. A more non-directive approach (maybe one that focuses more on how they feel rather than what they do) would leave most of the parents still in the dark, feeling very, very dissatisfied.

The importance of the IFFT team's after-hours availability to the parents and the child cannot be overstated. We routinely have the opportunity to disrupt a developing crisis and the parents and the child both regularly (and very appropriately) make use of this. Parents consistently express gratitude for having this option. As clinicians, we are similarly grateful to have the opportunity to help when it's most needed, and it is very satisfying to see families reach out to us less and less often as the child or teen gets well.

If you're wondering what became of Maricela, the girl in her bedroom who had just hurt herself at the beginning of the previous chapter, we will turn our attention toward her now.

Chief Takeaways from Chapter 7

For Parents

- If your child or teen is hurting themselves, I know you must be terrified, but please know that in most cases self-harm is very treatable.
- Many times when kids hurt themselves or think about taking their life, it's less about depression or hopelessness and more about anger and impulsivity, often precipitated by a conflict or upset with a family member or a peer.
- Many kids who self-harm are made worse by interacting on a device with other kids who struggle with the same problem (an echo chamber).
- Trips to the ER and possibly placement into a psychiatric hospital can often be confusing and overwhelming for parents and children. It's good to educate yourself about what that process entails so you can navigate it as smoothly as possible.
- One of the key ingredients of successfully helping your child or teen who engages in self-harm is slowly returning them to normal, developmentally appropriate expectations. You'll need a therapist's help with this, but it absolutely needs to happen.

For Clinicians

- Distinguishing anger from depression is essential as it will help you stay focused on the clinical interventions most helpful to the child and their parents.
- Time spent on devices and who the child or teen is interacting with online is a major situational variable that is contributing to their self-harming behavior and negative moods, and it should be a focus of your clinical attention.
- It's useful to obtain a commitment at the start of treatment from the child or adolescent to reduce or ideally eliminate self-harm, and to touch upon this in every session.
- If you tell parents to take their child to the ER, it is really important that you educate them fully on what to expect.
- Building up a kid's "muscle" for tolerating and participating in conversations with both you and their parents about self-harm urges and events is an essential part of treatment.
- Consider and then disrupt possible "functional" aspects of the self-harm; i.e., incentives the child is operating under to maintain the behavior (for example, avoiding school, homework, or other responsibilities).

References

Cialdini, R. B. (2001, October). Harnessing the science of persuasion. *Harvard Business Review*. https://hbr.org/2001/10/harnessing-the-science-of-persuasion

Deisenhammer, E. A., Ing, C.-M., Strauss, R., Kemmler, G., Hinterhuber, H., & Weiss, E. M. (2009). The duration of the suicidal process: How much time is left for intervention between consideration and accomplishment of a suicide attempt? *The Journal of Clinical Psychiatry*, 70(1), 19–24.

Diamond, G. S., Diamond, G. M., & Levy, S. A. (2014). *Attachment-based family therapy for depressed adolescents*. American Psychological Association. 10.1037/14296-000

Kruglanski, A. (2022, May 25). A quest for significance gone horribly wrong – how mass shooters pervert a universal desire to make a difference in the world. *The Conversation*. https://theconversation.com/a-quest-for-significance-gone-horribly-wrong-how-mass-shooters-pervert-a-universal-desire-to-make-a-difference-in-the-world-183199

McBain, R. K., Cantor, J. H., & Eberhart, N. K. (2022). Estimating psychiatric bed shortages in the US. *JAMA Psychiatry*, 79(4), 279–280. 10.1001/jamapsychiatry.2021.4462

Richardson, B. G., Surmitis, K. A., & Hyldahl, R. S. (2012). Minimizing social contagion in adolescents who self-injure: Considerations for group work, residential treatment, and the internet. *Journal of Mental Health Counseling*, 34(2), 121–132. 10.17744/mehc.34.2.206j243468882617

Robbins, M. S., Turner, C. W., Alexander, J. F., & Perez, G. A. (2003). Alliance and dropout in family therapy for adolescents with behavior problems: Individual and systemic effects. *Journal of Family Psychology*, 17(4), 534–544. 10.1037/0893-3200.17.4.534

Wick, N. (2005, December). UW professor takes new approach to preventing suicide. *University of Washington Magazine*. https://magazine.washington.edu/feature/uw-professor-takes-new-approach-to-preventing-suicide/

8 Case Example of Treating Self-Harm

The Girl Who Wouldn't Stop Hurting Herself

This is the first of two case examples included in this book to illustrate the strategies, techniques, and interventions, that might typically be used when treating a child or adolescent with a serious mental health condition. In both case examples, I have masked the identifying information of the patient and family to protect their privacy. In every other respect, however, the details of what unfolded in the patient's treatment are just as they occurred. It's important to note too that I chose the particular case that follows not because it's unusual in any way. Rather, I feel this is a good illustration of a typical self-harming patient and how we generally approach treatment from a family-focused perspective.

"Maricela" is a 13-year-old female growing up in a two-parent, middle-class household. She has one older male sibling, age 15. Maricela's brother functions well and does not suffer from a mental health condition. Maricela's mother is employed in sales and her father is retired from the military. The parents describe Maricela as very strong-willed, much more so than her brother, and as a young child she was very stubborn and often prone to temper tantrums (a more difficult-to-parent temperament). Despite some upsets and challenges when she was younger, Maricela generally did well until she entered middle school at age 11. Her parents noticed that she spent more time in her bedroom on her phone or laptop, was generally less interactive with her family, and was more easily irritated than she had been in the past.

Her condition vastly deteriorated over the following year. When Maricela's parents first contacted our clinic inquiring about IFFT services, life at home with her had ground to a virtual halt. Other than leaving her house to go to school each day, she spent almost all of her time isolated in her bedroom. If her parents tried to enter her room, she would scream at them to get out, making it all but impossible to have any kind of conversation with her. Maricela was intensely angry with her parents (seething with anger, actually), but was generally unable to say why except that she felt she was treated differently from her brother. In many ways

DOI: 10.4324/9781003397366-11

this was true—because she was so stubborn and reactive, her parents adopted a stricter, less flexible way of interacting with her (bidirectional mutual influence) and withheld many of the privileges and freedoms that her brother enjoyed. Maricela, of course, didn't see it this way and, instead, believed her treatment to be unfair and her anger justified.

At one time, this was likely a very high-functioning family, but as mutual hostility and rigidity grew, this was no longer the case. (I will discuss this family's pre- and post-treatment family functioning scores in more detail at the end of this chapter.)

Maricela's self-harming behavior emerged during this time period. She would cut in secret, never letting her parents know this had occurred until they found the remnants of it, such as bloody tissues in her trash can, or see the cuts on her arms if her shirt sleeves had inadvertently pulled up. Maricela certainly wouldn't discuss the self-harm; if her parents tried to talk with her about it, she would tell them the cuts were from her cat or offer some other equally implausible (and unsatisfying) explanation, or worse yet she would tell them to "shut the fuck up" and leave her alone. Eventually, Maricela's parents stopped asking in order to avoid the inevitable conflict. Her parents describe what we often hear from most of our parents, i.e., that they felt they had to walk constantly on eggshells around her. Not just because she was so explosive, but they were also worried that any misstep might trigger another self-harm event. Consequently, as is often the case, they had virtually stopped any kind of meaningful parenting of her because when they tried to set a limit with her, it would result in more hostility and self-harm.

Maricela had trouble sleeping her entire life (a family trait on her father's side), but this became especially problematic during this time period. She had unrestricted, unmonitored access to her phone (as I've discussed previously, always a bad idea with a kid with a mental health problem), and so she was up late every night, well past the time the rest of the family was asleep. Her parents suspected she was communicating online with people who were not a good influence on her but they could not be sure, and Maricela refused to discuss what she was doing on her phone at night. On one occasion, they were notified by the parents of one of Maricela's friends that she was engaging in sexualized conversations with an adult male with whom she had connected, but when confronted about this Maricela said her friend was lying. Falling asleep so late at night meant that Maricela was very difficult to wake up in the morning, setting the stage for terrible, high-conflict mornings and mutual irritability throughout the day.

Things worsened when Maricela's mother walked into her bedroom and found her using a razor blade on her arms. Maricela ran to the bathroom and locked herself in, and her parents called 911. She was taken to the ER and held there, but only overnight. She was belligerent to her mother who had gone to the ER with her, but Maricela persuaded the hospital social worker it was safe to send her back home. This event only made the situation at home even more volatile.

On the advice of the hospital, Maricela's parents arranged for a Partial Hospitalization Program (several hours in a classroom-type setting focusing on mental health), but it was only offered virtually and Maricela refused to attend. Her insurance company also offered individual therapy, but that person could see her only once a month and, again, only virtually. Maricela refused this as well, her stated reason being, "Therapy doesn't work," which was obviously resistance but also, at least for her, a factually accurate statement.

This was about the time Maricela's parents reached out to us for help. In order for our clinic to bill our services to her insurance company, we needed authorization from them to do so, as we were not part of their network of providers. We requested authorization, but it was denied for reasons that were never fully articulated to us or to the family. (This particular healthcare company is notoriously difficult to work with and often refuses to authorize services outside of its own inadequate network, presumably as a cost-savings measure.) However, it did offer to send to the family's home an unlicensed and very green therapist-in-training, who advised Maricela's parents to "take everything out of her bedroom until she behaves." (An absolutely terrible idea any way you look at it.) Maricela's parents eventually filed a complaint with a state agency that challenged the insurance company's denial of our services. Thankfully, the denial was overturned and we could finally begin.

We didn't know Maricela very well yet, but based on what we did know, we were able to form some initial hypotheses as to what was likely going on.

It was clear that Maricela was a more difficult-to-parent kid than her sibling and her strong-willed temperament elicited a very different parenting style in response. I had come to learn a bit about her mother and father, and my sense of them was that they were both kind-hearted, loving people who had nothing but good intentions and great affection for their daughter. They most definitely reacted to Maricela's strong-willed nature in equally strong ways (too strong), but they had deep regrets for how they interacted with her as they recognized many of their responses were less than ideal. Many times when Maricela did something they didn't care for, like yelling at them, becoming disrespectful, breaking rules, and so forth, they would become equally hot and reactive in return, getting into screaming matches with her and over-relying on strict consequences that didn't work (and just made Maricela even angrier and more bitter). Again, her parents were good people, but they simply didn't know how to best respond to Maricela's temperament and subsequent challenging behaviors. They all became increasingly angry, resentful, and disconnected from each other, and Maricela then retreated into her bedroom as just about any kid would in that same situation.

We also hypothesized, correctly it seems, that whatever Maricela was doing in her bedroom, whomever she was communicating with on her phone or laptop, was contributing to all this in a significant way. Online communication with negative peers in this case was a massive situational variable that needed to be disrupted. I know from experience that lonely, unhappy, and disconnected kids gravitate to other lonely, unhappy, disconnected kids, and once in that echo chamber, each participant mutually reinforces the others' dysfunction. I had no doubt that Maricela was communicating with one or more peers who engaged in self-harm as well ("You understand me because you cut too"), and likely these other kids were also angry with their own parents for slights real or imagined. (I say "imagined" here not to be dismissive or disrespectful; rather, a growing virtual community of teenagers cite "parental abuse" as the cause of their mental health issues when no actual abuse appears to be occurring.)

So, neither Maricela nor her parents had any idea how they had got themselves into this awful place, and they certainly had no idea how to get themselves out of it. Fundamentally, they all still loved each other, but everyone was angry and miserable, and the self-harm added an additional layer of terror for Maricela's parents, making the stakes for all sky high.

This case started off with a bang. We knew that the first thing we needed to do was get a handle on Maricela's unrestricted, unmonitored use of her phone. This situational variable needed immediate disruption, or at least needed to be made a lot safer. It seemed very likely to us that Maricela was, in fact, communicating with one or more people (likely kids, but who knows?) late at night who were not a good influence. We started by asking the parents to install Bark on her phone (one of many available parental control software programs) so that they would be alerted to any messaging that was worrisome or problematic. Bark is a good choice in that it allows the child or teen some privacy since it only sends parents an alert and snippets of messages that contain certain key words, such as "suicide," "cutting," "overdose," etc.

The very first week after we started treatment, Bark sent Maricela's parents an alert saying she had messaged a friend indicating that she had stolen a bottle of ibuprofen from their bedroom (medications were kept locked up, but she got it anyway) and was keeping it in her bedroom. When they went into her room to ask her about this, Maricela denied having taken the bottle despite the message, but, on our advice, they searched her room (which made her very mad) and found the bottle and removed it. Besides me, there were two other clinicians assigned to this family, and so one of them spoke with Maricela to assess whether she could commit to safety or instead needed to go to the ER and possibly a psychiatric hospital. Maricela stated she was safe and so she remained at home. The next day, her parents found several bloody tissues in her bedroom trash can, and that same day Maricela showed her skills training therapist about 20 cuts on her arm she had made the night before (but again stated she was committed to safety). I have no doubt that if Bark had not been installed on Maricela's phone she could easily have died by suicide that night.

Of course, Maricela's online activity needed further disruption beyond just monitoring her exchanges. In a perfect world, we would have been able to encourage her parents to vastly limit the amount of time she spent on her devices, which would have had the added benefit of likely decreasing the amount of time she spent in her bedroom. We see this again and again—once parents are no longer competing with their child's device for their attention, kids will naturally start to wander out of their bedrooms in search of something to do, with their parents ready, willing, and able to be that something. As we've discussed already, just reducing device time alone has a positive impact on a child or teen's mood. *[Side note: My wife and I noticed our youngest daughter would be super grumpy the longer she spent on her laptop. We'd pull her off of it and within 10 minutes she turned into a normal human being again.]*

It's not a perfect world, however, and because self-harm was a serious concern, we did not feel it was safe to vastly reduce phone use so early in treatment lest we risk a self-harm event in response. However, in month two of treatment, we did recommend to Maricela's parents that they use their cell plan's parental control feature to automatically disable her phone at 10:00 every night. This seemed like a good mid-way step that was probably safe enough to implement early in treatment. I've found with teens that their most problematic (and scariest) device use occurs late at night, so an early shut-off would disrupt her late-night communications. In addition, since sleep was such a problem for Maricela (and the irritability brought on by not getting enough sleep), this might have the added benefit of getting her to bed much earlier. Maricela was not at all happy about her phone shutting off at 10:00, but no kid ever is, after they've become accustomed to so few limits on their device usage.

Also in month two of treatment, we focused on other ways to help improve Maricela's sleep. She was currently not taking any psychotropic medication, so that seemed like an obvious point of intervention for both her low mood and sleep issues. Maricela had been tried on an antidepressant some months before, but she reported not liking the side effects so she stopped taking it. We suggested the parents speak with Maricela's psychiatrist about a possible course of trazodone, an older antidepressant that isn't used much anymore for the treatment of depression but is often prescribed as a sleep aid. Maricela was open to this as well, but after a few weeks her parents discovered that she had just been spitting it out because she said it gave her a headache and "didn't work anyway." I had my suspicions about her stated reasons; I think it was more likely she just didn't want to take it as she was just fine with staying up late at night. Maricela's psychiatrist later tried another antidepressant but with the same result (she just refused to take it altogether this time). We all collectively agreed not to take a third run at medication, and, for the remainder of Maricela's treatment, she was medication-free (which I think is awesome).

It would be an understatement to say that Maricela was not crazy about the idea of therapy. Like many of the adolescents we treat, she was reluctant to participate, and I don't think her feelings on this changed much for the ten months or so that we worked with her. She would often complain to her parents about having to attend sessions, especially her individual and family therapy sessions in the office. We typically do the skills training sessions remotely, but Maricela's parents felt these would be much more effective in person and in the home. They called that one correctly, as Maricela ended up developing a better relationship with her skills therapist than she did with her individual and family therapist. One of the advantages of IFFT is that there are at least two individual therapists working directly with each patient, so if the connection to one isn't good for whatever reason, we can rely more heavily on the relationship built by the other therapist. About mid-way through Maricela's treatment, we pivoted and let go of the in-office family therapy sessions and just did sessions in the home, and this went reasonably well.

I stated at the beginning of this chapter that this case was fairly typical, which is true with the exception of one factor. While not uncommon for kids to be guarded early in therapy, they usually warm up to the idea after a few months and generally become full participants. Maricela was unusual in the sense that she never really warmed up, and while she would grouse to her parents about therapy on the day it was scheduled, when her therapist arrived at the house Maricela was pleasant to her and generally polite. However, she remained guarded for several months, revealing little about herself in session and generally minimizing the severity of her issues and behaviors. Maricela's therapist is exceptionally skilled at warming kids up—her style is to be playful, use humor and affirmations a lot, and she just generally comes across as really easy to talk to. (Her in-office family therapist is highly skilled too but there was something about the chemistry or situation that didn't work as well.) Very gradually over time, Maricela would do more talking of a personal nature, but she never fully opened up. Most of these sessions were focused on teaching her DBT skills. However, she never made use of any of them, likely because a lack of skills wasn't really her problem, for reasons we'll discuss shortly.

We learned long ago that despite what one might think, most kids who are not fully engaged in their treatment can still get well. Remember, we can't change a child's temperament, but we can certainly change the situational variables that have resulted in a worsening of their temperament-informed behaviors. We definitely prefer that kids come along for the ride, but we've learned that if we change the parents' responses to a large enough degree, and we successfully disrupt the situational variables that are negatively influencing the child, lo and behold—even really reluctant kids get substantially better.

One of the most important situational variables we changed with Maricela's family very early in treatment was to vastly alter how her parents responded to her on a day-to-day basis. We could not do much work with Maricela early on to reduce her irritability for a number of reasons. She was not fully invested in treatment, as I mentioned, and she was locked into a number of distorted beliefs that fueled her anger and resentment toward her parents. These included "my parents don't love me," "the way my parents treat me is unfair," "my parents mistreat me so they deserve it when I get mad," and "I deserve more privileges like my brother." Cognitive distortions can be addressed, for sure, but that's very hard for a therapist to do when the kid doesn't trust you or possibly doesn't even particularly like you yet.

Since addressing Maricela's cognitive distortions wasn't possible right now, that avenue of change was closed to our team. Instead, I made changing how Maricela's parents responded to her the focus of my work in my sessions with them. It was clear that I needed to disrupt the cycle of bidirectional negative influence, as well as the parents' high reactivity to Maricela's disrespectful, oppositional behavior. So, I couldn't change her yet, but I could certainly try to change them.

The very first concept we discussed was "mirroring and matching," which again is a normal human tendency for people in conflict to *mirror* the other person's emotional state (if they get mad, you get mad), and *match* the person's pace, volume and intensity as they speak. This occurs in every argument I have ever observed (and it occurs in movies too, which I think is very cool). It's just what people in conflict often do. Most conversations will usually start off slowly, more softly, and in an emotionally well-regulated way (not always, of course, sometimes people just light up fast). As the conflict unfolds, however, one person invariably starts to speak in a louder voice, at a faster pace, and sharpens their tone of voice. Recall that moods and behaviors are contagious, so the other person begins to adopt the new pace, volume, and intensity. As a result of mirroring and matching, arguments unfold in a step-wise fashion, resulting in increased upset on both sides, often ending up with everyone yelling at each other, interrupting, and not even trying to understand the others' perspectives. It is important to note that all of this occurs unconsciously—no one knows that they're doing it, but we all do it.

In the case of Maricela and her parents, this type of heated pattern became the norm, and inevitably they reached a point in which there was very little communication occurring at all. Neither side saw the point—Maricela came to believe her parents were unreasonable and didn't listen, and they came to believe she was so irritable that she was impossible to talk to, and, of course, each person's views on this are at least partially true. The problem, however, is that no one is talking to each other, issues are never resolved in a reasonable way, there are no parental limits being set on Maricela's behavior (all aspects of healthy family functioning), and Maricela herself is being driven further into her negative beliefs about not being loved.

I've learned that there are ways to effectively disrupt this pattern of mirroring and matching in families. The first step is to describe the pattern to parents so that they have a new awareness of it, which they can then use to their advantage. You can't change a behavior if you don't know what the behavior is that needs changing. The second step is to identify the new behavior. If raising your voice with your child doesn't work and just provides them with incentive to raise their voice in return, what does work? Why, the opposite of course. You can use the principle of mirroring and matching to your own advantage by capitalizing on the reverse of it. This requires parents to go "low and slow," i.e., making a conscious effort not to match their child if they become more elevated, and, instead, staying matter-of-fact and remaining calm during a conversation that could lead to conflict. A lot of other professions have dialed into this concept as well. For example, teachers don't get into screaming matches with their students (usually). They briefly say what needs to be said, firmly if necessary, but not in an angry way, and then they quickly end the conversation. Nurses, flight attendants, and many other professions are the same way—matter-of-fact (but firm sometimes), no matter how elevated the other person might become.

In the case of Maricela's parents, this meant not ever raising their voices with her, no matter how irritable or disrespectful she was with them. Doing so would simply make matters much worse and often did. It took them a while to get the hang of staying matter-of-fact, but they embraced the concept fully right from the start, as they felt very guilty for all of the times in the past when they had raised their voices (as most parents do, in my experience).

Along with staying matter-of-fact with Maricela when she became upset, I also asked them to never (ever) speak with her when she was saying extremely angry and unkind things to them (talking to an angry kid who is respectful is obviously fine). This is a common mistake I see parents make, staying in a conversation with an angry, dysregulated, often accusatory teenager. It's problematic for numerous reasons, but primarily because it's too easy for the parent to become upset by something the kid is saying (usually the parent is being blamed or criticized), and then the conversation rapidly goes downhill from there. In addition, when someone is that angry, they are not thinking clearly and only communicating from an emotional place, which is rarely productive or helpful. Staying engaged with a very angry, disrespectful child or teen also sends the message to them that what they're saying, and the manner in which they're saying it, is a legitimate form of communication. There is nothing legitimate about a teenager screaming at you to "go fuck yourself." I encourage parents to say "I can't have a conversation with you when you're yelling at me, but I'd be happy to talk once you've calmed down" or, alternatively, "Dial that back please and we can talk, otherwise I'm walking away." Disengaging from an angry, disrespectful child or teenager is one of the single, most helpful strategies a parent should learn and implement. Talking to a kid who is yelling at you (and worse, a parent yelling back) not only doesn't work, it doesn't give them a chance to practice the skills needed to resolve conflict peacefully and respectfully. Once the child or teen has calmed down, parents can move back in again and tackle whatever the issue is when the kid is in a more reasonable frame of mind.

So, that's how we started with Maricela's parents—asking them to stay matter-of-fact and calm during moments of conflict, never to speak to her when she's highly upset and disrespectful or accusatory, and to re-engage with her only when she's calmed down. At least partially, this "flips the script" on her, meaning that it becomes harder for Maricela to hold onto the belief that her parents don't love her when they consistently speak to her in a way that isn't angry. And my goodness, Maricela's parents caught on to this fast. They took this to heart from day one and made an immediate shift in their behavior—staying matter-of-fact, going low and slow, not matching her intensity, and only staying engaged in conversation with her when she was being respectful. I do not recall one time over the course of their treatment where they messed up on this, which is remarkable and a testament to how much they love their daughter and want to help her.

These were the foundational skills we taught to Maricela's parents, and while necessary for them (necessary for all families, in fact), these skills alone weren't sufficient to entirely change Maricela for the better, nor were they expected to be.

On the seventh week of treatment, Maricela took another bottle of ibuprofen, this time from her parents' car. She denied having taken it and also refused to let her parents search her bedroom. She was again taken to the ER, and again she was not hospitalized because she committed to safety. Even though in IFFT we work hard to keep kids out of the hospital, we would have preferred that, in this instance, Maricela had been placed in a psychiatric hospital as it was her second, and what could have been fatal, overdose attempt. We did not have the opportunity to speak with the ER social worker, so we had to make do with the situation.

Despite the theft of the ibuprofen, we started to see some signs of improvement. Maricela was spending less time in her bedroom and more time around her parents. Not a lot more but some, and many of those interactions were positive or at least neutral. By this point, Maricela's parents were interacting with her much differently, which I suspect made it easier and more appealing for Maricela to emerge from her bedroom and spend time with them. Additionally, while she still didn't care much for family therapy, she was beginning to share more with her individual therapist.

We also encouraged the parents to start gradually resuming some reasonable limit setting with Maricela as they had completely backed off from that. As I've mentioned, it is very common for parents to fall into that pattern with a self-harming child, but I believe ultimately not setting fairly normal limits with a child or teen makes things infinitely worse. This is a very important point when it comes to understanding how to best help a child with a serious mental health condition. I feel all kids need parental limits, including kids who are depressed, anxious, and suicidal. When a parent stops telling their child, "That's not okay," especially if the child has grown up in a family environment that did set limits previously, they find this very odd and confusing. It never used to be okay to rage at their parents but now somehow it is? They must ask themselves why no one is stopping them from doing things that are obviously not okay.

Human beings are creatures of power. We like it when we have it and we absolutely do not like it when someone tries to take it away from us. It's normal and expected for parents to be "parental," to set limits with their kids when needed, but to do so in a fair, gentle, but reasonably firm way. When parents stop being parental, things in families go haywire and when kids get a taste of power (doing as they please), they run with it and heavily resist giving up that power once they experience it. This doesn't make them bad kids—it's just what kids do in that situation. And when parents let go of that power, it's not because they're bad parents, it's because they're scared to death that something terrible will happen.

With Maricela then, how did we safely return a reasonable amount of power to her parents so that they could start calling her out on some of her behavior that wasn't okay? And my belief is that in her heart she wanted to be called out because she knew no one else in her family would get away with speaking to her parents the way she did.

Maricela's parents had already regained some control over her phone in that they could shut it off remotely if needed, and they were disabling it at a reasonable time at night. We moved from this to leveraging her phone as a way to directly target her disrespect ("Dial that back please or I'm going to turn off your phone until you've spoken to me in a nicer way for a while."). Note that "a while" usually just needs to be a few hours, rarely much longer. Eventually, we added task completion as an expectation as well, such as straightening her room when asked or getting up on her own in the morning to an alarm on school days. What was interesting about Maricela is that her parents rarely had to actually shut off her phone—the mere mention of it alone was sufficient, which is certainly not the case with all kids.

By month three of treatment, Maricela's parents were reporting noticeably less irritability. Bark also picked up an exchange with a positive friend in which Mariela said, "Self-harm is stupid. I don't know why I do it." Interestingly as well, without telling anyone, she was using an app that tracked the number of days she had gone without a self-harm event, which she would quietly reset to zero after an incident. She started to become more playful with her parents and they with her (positive resonant exchanges). Maricela and her mother were also spending increased amounts of time together. Maricela's mother was quite handy and the two of them worked on a home-remodeling project together. On one occasion, the parents were away from home and just prior to their return Maricela cleaned up the entire house unprompted, something that would have been unheard of just a couple of months prior.

However, Maricela wasn't quite done yet with the self-harm. During month five of treatment, Bark sent another alert picking up a thread of texts that indicated she had broken back into the locked medicine cabinet and this time took a variety of medications, any one of which could have been fatal. Back to the ER, but this time our team and her parents felt it was necessary for Maricela to go to a psychiatric hospital. However, this was not just for her safety. We had other things in mind as well.

We have learned that placement in a psychiatric hospital can be used very strategically to disrupt a situation in which a patient's motivation to reduce self-harm is low. At the start of treatment, Maricela's stated commitment level to reducing or eliminating self-harm was only a 5 (10 being very committed), which we suspected was playing a role in all this. Furthermore, we had not yet fully disrupted her online activity with less-than-desirable peers. A hospitalization, when managed carefully, can be used very effectively to target what in this case appeared to be some lingering and situational variables, as well as a way to increase a patient's motivation to reduce self-harm.

I don't think Maricela was expecting to go to a psychiatric hospital, as she'd been in the ER before and it had never happened. It was also her first hospitalization and she had no idea what to expect, but within a day of arriving, she began calling her parents making demands that they come and get her, not knowing of course that it was not their decision to make. I was in very close contact with her parents (we spoke several times by phone and exchanged dozens and dozens of text messages over several days). On my advice, the parents were also in close contact with Maricela's treating psychiatrist at the hospital, and together we arrived at a strategy. It was clear early on that Maricela badly wanted to come home, which we used to our advantage. In fact, had she actually wanted to be in the hospital, or was enjoying her experience there (which is sometimes true with adolescents), the plan we devised never would have worked, nor would we have attempted it. We had two strategic goals—the first was to increase Maricela's motivation to stop hurting herself, and the second was to further place her parents back in a parental (power) role.

As I mentioned, Maricela started calling her parents immediately, and she not only made demands that they come to get her, but she was very angry with them and blamed them for her being there in the first place ("It's your fault I'm here"). I advised them to always take her calls (there were generally multiple calls per day), but if she became rude or disrespectful, to cue her just once ("Hey, not okay to talk to me that way"), and if she persisted to politely end the call and hang up. We knew Maricela badly wanted to get out, so her motivation to engage her parents in a way that would result in that happening was high. When she saw that demanding didn't work (this took several phone calls), she started to become more reasonable and respectful, albeit barely at first. The very worst thing her parents could have done would have been to stay on the phone while she was demanding things of them, or blaming them for being in the hospital. Any attempts to reason with her would have been futile and would only reinforce her belief that talking to her parents that way was acceptable. Getting Maricela into a place where she would listen and not blame was step one in the process, and that occurred fairly quickly.

Step two was ratcheting up Maricela's motivation to take self-harm more seriously and put her in a frame of mind to actually do some work on it (most of the time in session she would deny, minimize, "forget," blame her parents, and show no interest in learning DBT skills). Once Maricela became more respectful on the phone, I advised her parents to raise the topic of self-harm with her, and the conversation flowed as follows:

Maricela (M): Okay, okay, I'll be nice. I'm not yelling now.
Parent (P): Thank you. It's so much easier to have a conversation this way.
M: So, when are you taking me out? I want to go home today.

P: Well, there are some problems with that. First, it's not our decision to make. Once you're there, it is the hospital's decision as to when you go home. That's just how the whole thing works.

M: What do I need to do for them to decide that?

P: Well, being safe there I guess. Not just saying you are, but behaving in a way that shows them that you really are safe.

M: I've been doing that. But you could tell them I'm safe, right? That you think it's okay for me to come home now?

P: How am I going to do that?

M: What do you mean, how? You just do it.

P: Yeah but the thing is, I'm not convinced it is safe to take you home. Not at all in fact.

M: (Now getting angry) WHAT DO YOU MEAN? I TOLD YOU I'M SAFE!

P: Look, if you're going to yell at me, I'll say good-bye to you here and we can talk another time.

M: No! Okay I'm not yelling. Why can't you tell them I'm safe? Cause I am, I promise.

P: Because honestly, I don't think you are. I think as soon as you come home you're going to hurt yourself again. This is the third time you've taken pills. And each time you deny having done it, get mad at us, and tell us it's our fault. And you're still cutting and not talking about that to us or your therapist. So, no I don't think you're safe.

M: It is your fault! And what I do is none of your business!

P: We've made mistakes as parents, that's true. We've been hard on you not because we don't love you, but because we didn't know what to do. We've been working on that and are trying to do it differently, even if you don't see it that way. And it is our business, again, whether you see it that way or not. So no, I'm not going to bat for you with the hospital until something changes.

M: Like what?

P: Some reasonable commitment to safety. A real commitment, not a pretend one to get out. And if you don't want to do that, that's your decision, I'll leave it up to the hospital to decide when you can come home. But when they ask me my opinion, as of right now, I'm telling them you're not ready.

And just like that Maricela hangs up on her mom.

But that's okay, *package delivered*. They needed to step into it with her and hit the issue head-on in a way she never would have tolerated at home. She's in a safe place, and she's highly motivated, the perfect time to be direct and honest with her to effect positive change.

So this conversation, or variations on it, played out several more times in close proximity. Maricela tried various ways to keep turning things around on her parents, but they didn't give an inch and stood their ground. And it worked—in each conversation, she softened a little, became more genuine, and committed to working on things, and by the very last call, she was agreeable and soft with them. Maricela relented and her parents were back in the power position. *She leaned into them as a result*. And once she did, her parents immediately leaned back in return: *"We're calling your doctor right now. It's time for you to come home."*

Thankfully, the treating psychiatrist at the hospital went along with the plan as Maricela's parents had requested. Maricela asked him many times during her stay when she could leave, and his response each time was "What do your parents think of that idea?"

This was Maricela's first and last stay in a psychiatric hospital, And to the best of our knowledge, the last time she ever engaged in self-harm.

While Maricela was in the hospital, her parents learned that while she was being driven to the ER, she was texting a negative peer who told her, "Next time you grab a bottle of pills, I want some too." We locked down Maricela's devices even further after the hospitalization—she was given only a limited time on her phone each day (assuming the day went well), her negative peers were blocked, and she was prohibited from being on any type of social media.

One more event, which took place after the hospitalization, was significant for this family. A month or so after her discharge, Maricela woke up in an irritable mood, refused to go to school, and was very disrespectful. Her mother shut off her phone (after a warning), which made Maricela very angry. However, her mother did a great job and stood her ground, remained matter-of-fact, and refused to re-engage with Maricela until she spoke to her in a nicer way. It took Maricela some time (a couple of hours), but she eventually stopped demanding her phone, softened, and started crying, likely the first time she allowed herself to be vulnerable for who knows how long. Her mother leaned in right away and was equally soft in return. They were able to have a genuine, peaceful, respectful conversation about missing school and identifying what a preferable alternative would have been rather than simply refusing to go (asking in a nice way if she could just take the day off from school for no other reason other than feeling like she just needed it). Prior to treatment, this same event would have resulted in a heated argument, much more disrespect, Maricela isolating in her bedroom, and possibly self-harm.

Things between Maricela and her parents just got better and better from there. She slowly earned more time on devices in exchange for respectful behavior, and her social media was gradually returned to her (over a period of months). Overt disrespect ("I hate you!" or "You're stupid!") was gradually eliminated altogether, and what replaced it was only fairly typical teenage irritability on occasion. Maricela became much more loving and playful with both her parents and her brother, spent significantly more time out of her bedroom, and less time on devices when she was in there. She and her parents routinely started to say, "I love you" again after not having said it for almost two years. Maricela and her mother continued to do more projects around the house together. She and her father went to the gym each week and did a weight-lifting routine together. Both parents were also able to have many heart-to-heart conversations with her about events in the past. Although Maricela's therapist was able to do some cognitive restructuring around her beliefs that she was unloved, her thinking on this gradually changed all on its own, as everyone was now behaving in a loving way.

As Maricela started to improve, we gradually began to reduce the frequency of her sessions. We eventually let go of her family therapy sessions, as those seemed the least helpful for her. We continued the individual therapy sessions with her skills trainer in the home for some time (by this point they were every other week) until Maricela felt she no longer needed those. At this point, we were just down to my parent sessions every other week until Maricela's insurance company abruptly and without explanation decided to no longer authorize our services. (Boo!)

Clinical Outcomes

In IFFT, we routinely measure and track patient and family outcomes, both at the start of treatment, at a mid-way point, and at the time services are discontinued. We want to make sure that the treatment we are providing is actually being helpful and to what degree. There are various schools of thought on how to go about this, but our clinic uses two measures.

The first is the Youth Outcomes Questionnaire (Y-OQ2.01), a 64-item inventory completed by parents that measures the degree of distress experienced by a child or teen, as well as progress in treatment based on changes in the severity of presenting problem behaviors (Wells et al., 1999). The Y-OQ is a well-established instrument, and it is a commonly used mental health outcomes measure. The measure produces a total score, with higher scores indicating a greater degree of clinical and behavioral impairment. A total score of 47 or greater is considered the clinical cutoff (the child has significant problems), and the goal of treatment is to reduce that score as close to the normal range as possible (the community, or nonclinical sample,

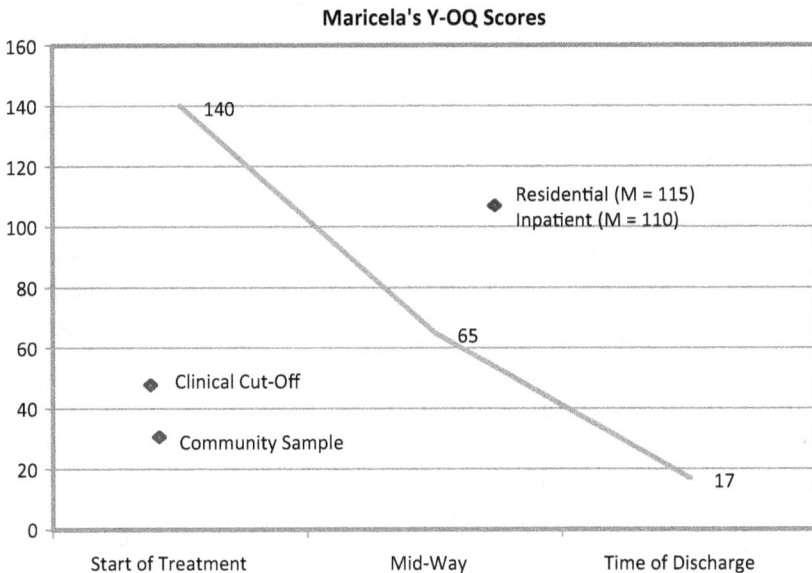

Figure 8.1 Maricela's scores on the Y-OQ at intake, mid-way through treatment, and at the time of discharge.

of 23.3 or less). The average total score of children and teens in inpatient (hospital) settings is 110, and for kids in residential treatment programs, it is 115.

Maricela's Y-OQ scores over the course of treatment can be seen in Figure 8.1.

Note how high Maricela's Y-OQ scores were at the start of treatment (140). This is well above the mean (average) scores of children and teens in residential treatment and inpatient programs (115 and 110 respectively). By the mid-way point in treatment, her score had dropped to 65, but this is still above the clinical cut-off of 47, so there was still work that needed to be done. At the conclusion of treatment, Maricela's Y-OQ score had dropped to a remarkably low score of 17, which is well below the average score of kids without mental health problems.

The second outcome measure used in our clinic is the Child & Adolescent Family Functioning Inventory (Sunseri, 2022). The CAFFI is based on my research, which, as I've mentioned, shows a relationship between how well a family functions and the severity of the child's mental health condition. It is a brief (25-item) measure of family functioning along five domains: Ability to Solve Problems, Managing Stress and Conflict, Closeness and Connection, Effective Communication, and Other

Relational Subsystems (school, siblings, and peers). The CAFFI is completed by the parents, and scores reflect their perceptions of how well their family functions within these domains. Higher scores on the CAFFI indicate poorer family functioning. The scores obtained on the CAFFI are then compared to a normative (nonclinical) sample, with the goal of treatment to lower the family's scores as close to the normal range as possible. I have made the CAFFI publically available at no cost to other clinics that might wish to use it (see the article I referenced above for a link to download the CAFFI).

Maricela's five CAFFI scores over the course of treatment (Intake, Mid-Way, and Time of Discharge) are compared to a normative sample in Figure 8.2.

Maricela's three total scores over the course of treatment in comparison with the normative sample are shown in Figure 8.3.

As can be seen, all five of the family's subscale scores decreased (improved) over the course of her treatment. In fact, by the time her case was closed, all of her subscale scores, as well as her total score, were well below the normative sample (better than the nonclinical sample).

This was a wonderful family to work with in so many ways. Maricela's parents were deeply caring people and they were highly committed to helping her in any way possible. Their openness to working on ways to change their behavior for the better made our jobs so much easier. As they

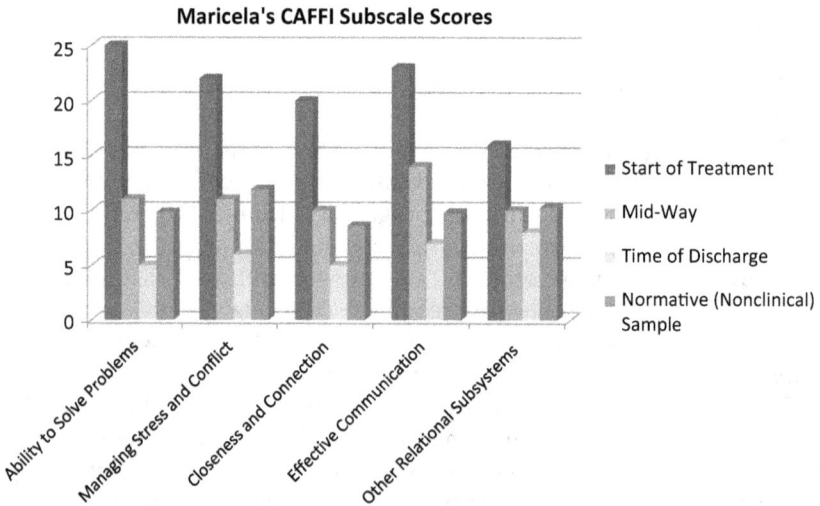

Figure 8.2 Maricela's scores on the five CAFFI subscales at intake, mid-way through treatment, and at the time of discharge in comparison to a normative (nonclinical) sample.

Maricela's CAFFI Total Scores

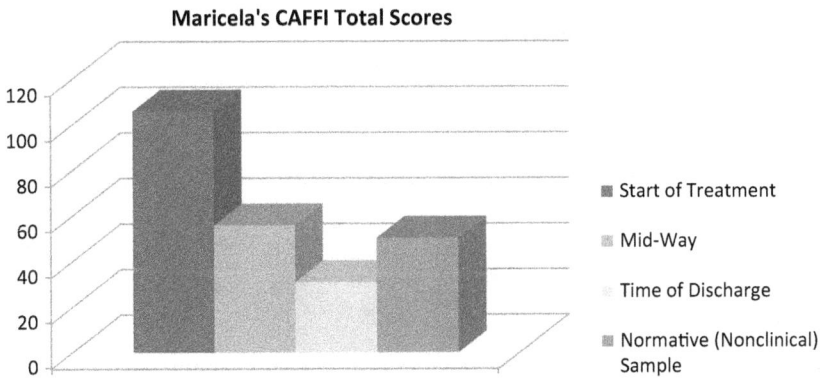

Legend:
- Start of Treatment
- Mid-Way
- Time of Discharge
- Normative (Nonclinical) Sample

Figure 8.3 Maricela's total scores on the CAFFI at intake, mid-way through treatment, and at the time of discharge in comparison to a normative (nonclinical) sample.

became less reactive and more matter-of-fact in the face of Maricela's anger and disrespect, it became increasingly difficult for her to maintain the belief that she was unloved by them. This change in their dynamic was probably the single most important ingredient that led to Maricela's improvement. As reactivity and bad feelings were reduced, and as warmth and connection increased, it allowed Maricela to gradually emerge from her bedroom and actually seek out positive interactions with both of her parents. The connection to her negative peers was severed, and so Maricela was no longer influenced by them to hurt herself. All of this combined allowed her parents to step back into a parental role and set reasonable limits and expectations around her behavior, something that all kids want and desperately need from their parents.

Maricela is a great kid with great parents. She just drifted off course for a while and needed a little help from her family to find her way back.

References

Sunseri, P. A. (2022). The child and adolescent family functioning inventory (CAFFI): Development and psychometric properties. *Journal of Psychology and Psychotherapy*, *12*(1): 1–7. DOI: 10.35248/2161-0487-22.12.423.

Wells, M. G., Burlingame, G. M., & Lambert, M. J. (1999). Youth outcome questionnaire (Y-OQ). In M. E. Maruish (Ed.), *The use of psychological testing for treatment planning and outcomes assessment* (pp. 497–534). Lawrence Erlbaum Associates Publishers.

Part III

Treating Social Isolation and Anxious Avoidance

9 Anxious Avoidance

Prevalence, Evidence-Based Treatments, and the Role of Family and Situations

> *Lucas is a transgender 17-year-old male who has been diagnosed with generalized anxiety disorder and major depressive disorder. He is also slowly being erased from existence. Lucas's father is furious with him because despite seeing the same therapist for three years, Lucas once again forgot there was a Zoom session today and seems altogether unconcerned that his family has to pay for the session anyway. Lucas has dropped out of high school, almost never leaves the house, does not bathe or brush his teeth, and passes almost the entire day on his laptop. Lucas's parents understand he has a mental health condition and they are trying very hard to be compassionate, but they also feel powerless and have given up hope. All pleas from his parents to engage in life, in any capacity, are met with "You know I can't do that." If pressed to do something, Lucas will become explosive, and he'll scream at his parents, telling them they are to blame for his misery.*

Perhaps one of the most prevalent consequences of the onset of the COVID-19 pandemic and the social isolation that ensued is a wave of children and adolescents who have developed profound social anxiety that has persisted even as the restrictions of the pandemic have gradually lifted. This ranges from mild social avoidance, such as a general reluctance to re-engage fully with peers and family, to almost complete avoidance of life in general. It is not uncommon for adolescents to present for treatment (or more accurately, to have been presented for treatment by their parents) who spend almost all of their time in their bedroom, rarely interacting with family, minimally participating at school, or not attending at all, and sometimes not even taking care of their basic hygiene. Parents typically become paralyzed in this situation because when the child is asked to try to do something, anything really, they are met with tremendous resistance and countless arguments from the child or teen as to why they are incapable of

DOI: 10.4324/9781003397366-13

doing what is asked of them, no matter how slight. Parents become caught between two competing positions—desperately wanting their child to fully re-engage in life, but also trying to remain understanding and compassionate as they bear witness to their child's profound suffering.

It is important to note that highly avoidant teens and young adults predate the onset of COVID-19 and have existed for some time. For example, in Japan, it is estimated that as many as a million adolescents and young adults refuse to leave their bedrooms, sometimes for a decade or longer (Kremer & Hammond, 2013). The word used to describe these young people is "hikikomori," which is well-known in Japan. Not surprisingly, given what we know about social contagion, once the hikikomori started to draw national attention (there is a novel and comic book about the condition), the prevalence of it began to increase. One such person described his experience as follows:

"I had all kinds of negative emotions inside me," he says. "The desire to go outside, anger towards society and my parents, sadness about having this condition, fear about what would happen in the future, and jealousy towards the people who were leading normal lives." (Kremer & Hammond, 2013)

Thankfully, as is the case with self-harm, anxious avoidance is quite treatable, including in very extreme cases like Lucas. In this chapter, we will start by looking at the prevalence of anxious-avoidant behavior in children and teens, and try to understand why it's become so common post-COVID. (Hint: As you might guess by now, there's much more to it than just COVID). We will consider the situational/contextual variables that provide the incentive for both the development of this condition and the maintenance of the avoidant behaviors over time. We will take a look at the most well-established, evidence-based model of treatment for anxiety, but also discuss the ways that treatment needs to be modified and implemented for it to be successful in patients with very serious anxiety and avoidant conditions. In the next chapter, I will provide a detailed, highly effective family-focused approach to successfully treating extremely anxious children and adolescents such as Lucas, whose lives have been severely diminished but who still have the potential to make a full recovery.

Anxiety in Children and Adolescents

Feeling anxious from time to time is a regular part of life. Adolescents might sometimes feel worried about family issues, friends, or school-related stressors. The difference between an anxiety disorder and occasional, common anxiety is that "for people with an anxiety disorder, the anxiety does not go away and can get worse over time. The symptoms can interfere with daily activities such as task performance, schoolwork, and relationships" (NIMH, n.d.). When evaluating anxiety symptoms, it is important to consider their severity, persistence over time, and impact on the person's quality of life. There are various kinds of anxiety disorders, including phobia-related disorders (fear of something specific such as a fear of flying), social anxiety disorder (nervousness around other people), panic disorder (characterized by panic or anxiety attacks), and generalized anxiety disorder (excessive worry about everyday things) (NIMH, n.d.).

During adolescence, anxiety is usually related to social approval, appearance, and issues around independence (American Academy of Child and Adolescent Psychiatry [AACAP], n.d.). Of course, there are countless other reasons why teenagers experience anxiety, which under-scores how crucial it is to navigate everyday life issues and learn to cope with them. Anxiety may present in many different ways, such as "ex-cessive fears and worries, feelings of inner restlessness, and a tendency to be excessively wary and vigilant ... feelings of continual nervousness or extreme stress ... dependent, withdrawn, or uneasy" (AACAP, n.d.). Physical symptoms may include body pains, fatigue, discomforts related to puberty, hyperventilation, blotching, flushing, sweating, trembling, and being easily startled.

Prevalence Pre- and Post-COVID-19

Comparisons of depression and anxiety among children and adolescents pre- and post-pandemic report significant increases in anxiety and depression levels, especially for females (Hawes et al., 2022; Wang et al., 2022). A meta-analysis (a type of study that combines the results of multiple other studies) of depressive and anxiety symptoms in children and adolescents during COVID-19 indicates that global prevalence likely doubled during the pandemic (Racine et al., 2021).

The unprecedented nature of the pandemic meant families had prac-tically no point of reference for how to cope. Adolescence is typically a time of burgeoning independence, yet quarantines and stay-at-home orders around the world require teens to attend school online, miss out on social interactions with their peers, and spend much more time at home with their families (Lee, 2020, as cited in Lorenzo et al., 2021). The pandemic brought significant worries and concerns to parents as well, which likely brought with it some degree of emotional contagion in the family household. Research by Nicole Lorenzo and her colleagues at Florida International University suggests that the individual character-istics of each family member can influence their response to a serious life event such as COVID-19 and that parental anxiety and depression can affect their offspring not only in childhood but also through late adoles-cence (Lorenzo et al., 2021).

Evidence-Based Treatment for Children with Anxiety: Exposure Therapy

A well-established and effective method for treating anxiety is a form of cognitive behavior therapy (CBT) called exposure therapy (NIMH, n.d.). Exposure therapy has its origins in the behavior therapy movement of the 1950s, though the research during that time was mainly on adults (Abramowitz et al., 2011, p. 13). The first randomized controlled trials (RCTs) of exposure therapy in children took place during the late 1960s and early 1970s (Whiteside et al., 2020, p. 10). However, the earliest recorded exposure interventions for children actually took place in the 1920s with Mary Cover Jones, also known as "the mother of behavior therapy." In the 1990s, increased research on child anxiety disorders established the efficacy of exposure-based therapy for this young population and laid the groundwork for child anxiety treatment research today (Whiteside et al., 2020, p. 10).

Exposure therapy requires the therapist to "create a safe environment in which to 'expose' patients to the things they fear and avoid" (APA, 2017). When people avoid what scares them, the avoidant behavior provides short-term relief but can cause long-term problems by worsening the fear. A patient who chronically avoids anxiety-provoking situations has adopted an anxiety-reduction strategy, but, paradoxically, it is this very strategy that perpetuates and exacerbates their anxiety over time.

Thus, exposure therapy aims to help people confront the underlying fears that prevent them from engaging in activities they typically avoid, as well as teach them how to tackle new fears and anxieties as they progress through life (NIMH, n.d.; Southam-Gerow, 2019). Exposure therapy helps through decreased reactions to fears over time (habituation); weakens associations between fears and bad outcomes (extinction); provides proof that the person can face their fears and successfully manage their anxiety (self-efficacy); and creates new, more fact-based beliefs about the experience of fear (emotional processing) (APA, 2017).

Resistance to Exposure Therapy

Active and willing participation of the patient is necessary for the best results from exposure therapy, but many teens refuse to tolerate the short-term spike in anxiety that results from this treatment (Foa & Andrews, 2006). From the perspective of the child or teen, however, avoidance makes perfect sense. As adults, we can see the value of pushing through hard things, and while kids may understand the rationale (and perhaps even the science) of exposure therapy, that doesn't mean they'll actually be willing to engage in it (far from it in many cases). It is much easier and more comfortable to continue to avoid, and my goodness, avoid they do.

For highly avoidant teens like Lucas in our case example, it takes some very skillful clinical maneuvering to make this happen.

Creativity and persistence are essential when therapists encounter resistance from teens in treatment (Bennett et al., 2017). The therapist must work hard at building a therapeutic alliance, understand the teen and their strengths, and communicate in a way that is therapeutic rather than stigmatizing. Exposure therapists must be able to adapt their approach on the fly and dial any given exposure intervention up or down depending on the client's needs (Southam-Gerow, 2019, p. 133). This way, if the patient is reluctant to engage in an exposure task, the therapist can pivot to discussing alternatives they already have in mind. Empathy, humor, and a down-to-earth, genuine approach are all helpful for easing resistance to therapy (Peris et al., 2020).

An Example of Exposure Therapy

Take, for example, a teenager with a fear of swimming. They might refuse to learn how to swim because of fear they might drown. As a result, they never join family or friends when they go to the swimming pool or the ocean, and they end up missing out on spending time and making memories with them. Their fear of swimming is essentially kept alive and made more powerful each time the teen avoids an opportunity to swim. Furthermore, the child's fear of swimming becomes part of the family story, repeated for years, and accepted as fact ("Oh we all know Pedro is too afraid to swim").

Here are a few different examples of how exposure therapy might be paced with a patient:

Graded Exposure

A therapist would help Pedro formulate an exposure fear hierarchy in which he ranks his fears according to difficulty (APA, 2017). Mildly difficult exposures come first, before moving on to more challenging ones. Being in an actual swimming pool is currently too scary for Pedro, so graded (gradual) exposure might look something like this for him: 1) Imagine yourself standing in the shallow end of a swimming pool, with your head above the water. 2) Imagine holding onto the edge of the pool and dipping your head underwater for a few seconds. 3) Imagine treading water in the deep end of the pool where your feet cannot touch the ground. 4) Go to a swimming pool and spend five minutes wading in the shallow end. 5) Go to a swimming pool for ten minutes and practice holding your breath underwater while still holding on to the pool's edge. 6) Spend 20 minutes in the swimming pool to practice being in the water and holding your breath. 7) Enroll in a swimming lesson. 8) Attend the swimming lesson. Obviously, this approach is likely to be very effective if Pedro is highly motivated to learn how to swim, but as we shall see, many adolescents would never be willing to participate in this type of exposure plan. They definitely might want to learn how to swim, but not badly enough to override the initial increase in anxiety that such a plan entails.

Flooding

Unlike graded exposure, flooding begins with the most difficult tasks in the fear hierarchy (APA, 2017). Instead of imagining oneself in the swimming pool, a patient would start by just enrolling in and attending a swimming lesson, and tolerating the discomfort until it naturally begins to subside.

Systematic Desensitization

Sometimes, relaxation exercises can be combined with exposure to help manage anxiety and associate the fear with relaxation (APA, 2017). While breathing exercises would obviously be impossible underwater, this patient could take long, deep breaths while their head is above water. This would support them in being calmer and more relaxed as they face the fear of swimming.

Outcomes Research

A 2022 review by Alessandra Teunisse and her colleagues provides evidence for the efficacy of exposure to feared stimuli for young people aged 14–24 years. However, no randomized controlled trials (RCTs)—widely regarded as the "gold standard" for evaluating intervention effectiveness—specifically assess exposure for treating DSM-5 anxiety disorders (Teunisse et al., 2022). Stated another way, while exposure therapy is shown to be effective in treating anxious youth, more empirical studies are needed to close the current major gaps in knowledge.

Therapy format and social support are potential contributing factors to exposure therapy efficacy. Thomas Bertelsen and his colleagues at the University of Bergen in Norway developed a community-based group CBT program that included high degrees of exposure practice, family involvement, and school involvement (Bertelsen et al., 2022). Follow-up at 12 months showed that all outcomes were superior to other studies of the effectiveness of exposure therapy. This combination of group setting, heavy exposure practice, and family and school involvement shows promise for real-world application and treatment efficacy.

Research on "big avoiders" (avoiding not just one thing but many things) such as the case example of Lucas and many of the kids we treat with IFFT, is relatively sparse. Nevertheless, case studies do exist and provide valuable insight regarding exposure and adolescents. A 2019 case study by Alexander Tice provides an account of adapting exposure for a 14-year-old with obsessive-compulsive disorder (OCD) and comorbid anxiety disorder (Tice, 2019). "Daniel" suffered from severe anxiety to the point of significant functional impairment, and his main obsessions and compulsions were about contamination and washing. Daniel refused to go to school and avoided leaving the house, resulting in limited social interactions with peers. Over the course of a 25-session exposure treatment, Daniel successfully achieved his therapy goals: He had reduced levels of obsessions and compulsions, and improved functioning inside and outside the home (i.e., increased engagement in developmentally appropriate tasks and social activities). Practically speaking, the entire family was able to return to a more normalized lifestyle rather than having to work around Daniel's avoidance. Daniel was able to engage in the activities he previously avoided, such as going to crowded places, playing with friends, and eating in restaurants.

Situational and Contextual Variables That Incentivize and Maintain Avoidant Behavior

The vignette of Lucas at the start of this chapter is a pretty good example of the anxious-avoidant teenagers that my colleagues and I treat in our clinic. Obviously, no teen wakes up one morning as debilitated as Lucas. The process, however, unfolds gradually over time.

It's very much like the allegory of the frog in the pot of boiling water. As the story goes, if someone were to drop a frog in a pot of boiling water, it immediately jumps out. However, if instead, the frog is put in a pot of cold water, but the heat is gradually turned up to a boil, the frog will eventually perish. (I know it's a gross allegory, but it serves our purposes here.) I'm sure if a family of a psychologically healthy teen was told that one day the kid would wake up and stop going to school, no longer leave their bedroom, stop bathing or brushing their teeth, and pretty much appear miserable all of the time, they would think that couldn't possibly happen. The kid wouldn't believe it either. And, they'd be right, it doesn't happen that way, not on a single day—but slowly, by degrees, over several months or even years.

So how does it happen?

In my experience, it's a confluence of events, a perfect storm, if you will. Each of the following possible contributing factors seems to play some role in the development of anxious avoidance to varying degrees. Understanding each factor's role points us in the direction of how to disrupt and mitigate their contribution to the problem, thereby vastly improving the child's mental health and overall well-being.

I will go through each one of these factors, and once done, we'll turn our attention to what we do in treatment to address and mitigate each.

Temperament

Anxious-avoidant teens often seem to have been anxious-leaning young children. I have no real data to back this up other than this is what many parents tell me about their child. Every so often, I'll hear that a particular kid was not overly anxious in their younger years, but this is generally not the norm. That kids were more anxious relative to their siblings or peers makes sense to me when I meet an anxious teenager—to some degree the anxiety feels like a temperament issue, i.e., they likely came into the world running more on the anxious side.

I suppose instead of an anxious temperament, the child's present-day anxiety might be the result of some negative childhood experience, such as trauma for example. We know that physical, sexual, or emotional abuse can lead to the development of anxiety symptoms, so this of course does occur. While I have worked with many traumatized children, in most cases of anxious-avoidant teens, I often find no trauma history.

It stands to reason that a temperamentally anxious child would be more vulnerable to the development of later problematic anxiety as an adolescent. As we discussed in Chapter 1, it's not easy being a teenager in the 21st century, and an anxious-leaning kid is going to struggle more with day-to-day stress, especially in social experiences with more demanding performance-related challenges (grades, driving, and so on) than a temperamentally less anxious kid. So, some of the age-typical demands or expectations of being a teenager might be more challenging to them, but, as we'll see in just a bit, it's still very important that they be asked to meet and master those demands anyway.

The Principle of Least Effort

In Chapter 3, I discussed what is known as the Principle of Least Effort, which is highly relevant to understanding the anxious-avoidant child. The idea behind this is that there exists a tendency among animals, people included, when faced with multiple behavioral options, to choose the one that is least effortful. For example, and somewhat ironically, when I drive into the parking lot of my gym, I make every effort to find a parking space closest to the entrance.

Teenagers engage in making similar decisions when faced with a task that requires effort. And there's a lot of effort involved in a typical teen's life: Getting up early for school; spending six hours a day in a classroom learning about things that often aren't particularly interesting; doing even less interesting homework; taking care of chores at home (when chores are given that is); cleaning their room; engaging in sports; taking music lessons; working on their driver's license; getting a job; and so on. All of these age-typical responsibilities require sustained effort.

Unhelpful Reinforcement Patterns

If sustained, effortful behavior is difficult, and there is a natural human tendency to find solutions that are less effortful, one can easily see the potential for incentives to come into play in all the wrong ways. If a task or responsibility is avoided successfully, the strategies implemented to avoid those difficult tasks will have been reinforced, thereby strengthening the avoidant behavior. As I mentioned before, reinforcement can take place outside of the person's awareness, i.e., we don't have to know that our behavior is being reinforced for the principles of reinforcement to work.

Here's an example. It's not uncommon for kids to say they are too anxious to take a shower and so they avoid bathing. Sometimes, they'll say it's because seeing themselves in the mirror makes them anxious, or the feel of the water on their skin is uncomfortable. A reinforcement pattern begins to emerge that looks like this. Let's say a kid's objective is not to take a shower, either because it legitimately brings up anxious feelings, or, like many teenagers without anxiety, they just don't want to do it. It's actually pretty normative for late elementary school and early middle-school kids not to want to take baths and showers, so the origins of developing avoidance might often just start this way innocently.

When a child is reluctant to bathe, a parent will start by trying to talk to them about the importance of taking care of their hygiene. Parents typically make countless attempts to change their child's behavior (get them to take a shower) by trying to persuade them of the importance of doing so. (Remember, kids are not always rational actors, and arguments that might convince another adult of something often fall flat with kids.) Sometimes the child will agree with the parent and perhaps say they'll take a shower ("Yeah, yeah, I know, I will."), but days go by and nothing happens.

In this case, two aspects of the child's behavior have been reinforced: 1. they've learned that simply agreeing to their parents' request puts an immediate end to the uncomfortable conversation (agreement is negatively reinforced), and 2. they've learned that delaying buys them at least several days without having to take a shower and without another unpleasant conversation about it with their parents. From a kid's perspective, this makes total sense as an avoidance strategy—it got their parents off their back and they still managed to successfully avoid taking a shower.

Parents will often tell me their child or teen is lazy. They offer this up as a causal explanation for why their child doesn't engage in various age-appropriate responsibilities. I tell them their child is not lazy; they've just been reinforced for the wrong things. It's true of all of us: If avoidance is reinforced (it gets us out of doing something we don't want to do), we're all going to be far less likely to do those things. I'll confess something here of myself and it's not particularly flattering but it's completely true. I do not like emptying the dishwasher, so I avoid it at all costs. Unfortunately for my wife, she's reinforced me countless times for not doing it because I've learned that if I don't empty it she eventually will. I don't think that makes me lazy; I think it makes me someone who doesn't like emptying the dishwasher. My avoidant strategy works quite well for me, but not at all well for my wife. (Lest you think I'm a terrible husband, I'm pretty sure I make up for my dishwasher-avoidant tendencies in other many areas of our relationship. Hopefully, anyway.)

Okay, back to our example, here's what happens next. Parents almost always reach a point where they get super frustrated with the asking/persuading approach and the ongoing avoidance. Even the nicest of parents eventually move on to frustration and anger—raised voices, heated exchanges, and more commanding-type language ("Get in that shower NOW!").

You've come this far in the book so I think it's time to test your knowledge. What principles have I discussed so far that come into play when parents raise their voices and start barking out orders? And then what negative behavioral responses on the part of the child become incentivized and highly predictable? Answer: Raising one's voice invokes the principle of mirroring and matching. If a parent raises their voice and talks faster and more insistently, the child mirrors that back and matches their emotional intensity. Commanding-type language invokes the principle of tug-of-war: The more insistent a parent becomes to get a kid to do something, the more insistent a kid becomes that they are not going to do it.

The other thing a heated exchange does in this situation is to provide the kid with an incentive to come back with increasingly imaginative, persuasive arguments as to why they shouldn't do what's being asked of them. These arguments can often be very creative. The most convincing arguments tend to be those designed to elicit guilt and uncertainty in the parent. This is what that might sound like in the showering example:

Parent (P): Hey, so look, how many conversations about taking a shower have we had? It's something we all need to do in life.

Child (C): Why are we still talking about this? I told you taking showers makes me anxious.

P: We're still talking about this because you don't do it.

C: I said I would. Why don't you believe me?

P: No more promises. You need to take a shower today.

C: Okay but you have to let me do it when I'm ready. You know forcing me to do things doesn't work. It makes me want not to shower at all. Is that what you want?

P: You know that's not what we want.

C: If it's hard for me why do you want me to do it? Are you trying to make me more anxious? Why don't you understand what I need? I've told you over and over how bad it makes me feel and I'll do it when I'm ready.

P: I'm not trying to make you feel bad.

C: Well, you are, so stop. If you were better parents, you'd be handling this differently. Good parents would be more understanding and they don't force kids to do things that they can't do.

Oh, ouch. I bet that last one is the argument that would actually get traction and get most parents to back down. Parents are already feeling terribly guilty about having an anxious-avoidant kid who's paralyzed by life, so in the face of that comment I bet most of them would ease off, retreat from the discussion, and then second guess themselves for days ("Are they right? Maybe we are bad parents and need to be more understanding.").

These types of conversations occur countless times in families, sometimes over many years. The parent makes a request, the kid refuses, and the parent backs down. Rinse and repeat (and reinforce) over and over, so it's no wonder the avoidant behavior becomes firmly cemented in place.

A trauma therapist might look at shower anxiety through a trauma lens—maybe something happened to them in the shower? A DBT therapist might look at this as a skills deficit or a distress tolerance problem—what skills can the child be taught so they can tolerate taking a shower? In IFFT, we assess for both of these elements as well. But in most cases, as I mentioned, there is no trauma history that would account for the avoidance, and in my experience, many avoidant kids resist the use of skills. Then what?

My example so far has been about showering. This same logic—the path of least effort and inadvertently reinforcing avoidant behavior—applies to just about any other behavior common to anxious-avoidant kids: Not coming out of their rooms; minimally willing (and sometimes not willing at all) to leave the house; not spending time with immediate family and extended family; not going to school and/or not doing homework; being unwilling to do chores around the house; and total avoidance of big-ticket, developmentally normal responsibilities like getting a driver's license or a part-time job.

Let's keep looking at other situational variables in addition to unhelpful reinforcement patterns that incentivize and maintain anxious-avoidant behaviors.

Parental Style and the Need to (Over) Protect

We learned in Chapter 1 that for children to learn they are capable of handling difficult situations, it is crucial for them to take small, age-appropriate risks and be afforded opportunities to make decisions independent of their parents. It is normal for parents to want to step in and protect their children from suffering, but too much enabling behavior can be detrimental.

In her excellent TEDMED talk, psychologist Anne Marie Albano explains that when kids with anxiety escape and avoid challenging situations and get other people to do them for them, they become even more anxious and come to believe they are incapable of navigating age-typical situations (Albano, 2020). Albano gives examples of common behaviors in children with anxiety: Not wanting to go to school, worrying about being embarrassed in class, and difficulty making friends. For each of these behaviors, defining the opposite action (purposely stepping into an anxiety-provoking situation rather than avoiding) is essential. A question a person might ask themselves might be: What is the opposite of what my emotions are telling me to do? For example, if the child does not want to go to school due to difficulty making friends, an opposite action could be to go to school and strike up at least one brief conversation with a peer each day.

I highly recommend that both therapists and parents alike watch Albano's TED talk. I routinely ask parents who have an anxious-avoidant child to watch it, and we discuss it in our parent sessions. This is often very impactful for parents, especially when I have been unsuccessful in my efforts to persuade them to enable their children less and avoid rescuing them from everyday, age-appropriate, anxiety-provoking situations. A parent's desire to protect is understandable, but stepping in and shielding kids from whatever is making them anxious is the opposite of being helpful.

Researchers Lindsay Holly and Armando Pina at Arizona State University describe the "protection trap" that parents fall into, which includes allowing the child to avoid uncomfortable situations, telling the child what to do and say when they are anxious, or acting on behalf of the anxious child (Holly & Pina, 2015). An example of that would be ordering food for a child in a restaurant because they are "too shy" to speak to the server directly. While these reactions provide short-term relief to the child, they are not helpful for them in the long term and worsen their anxiety. These parents are typically not sabotaging their children on purpose; in fact, they generally do not make the connection that their constant stepping in to rescue their child actually increases the child's anxiety (Landro, 2013).

Instead, parents can help their anxious child by monitoring their own responses, giving positive attention when the child does face their fears, and minimizing the positive attention toward anxiety (e.g., providing less reassurance to the child because reassurance conveys that there is indeed a danger to worry about and/or that the child is not capable of successfully tolerating the feared experience).

Research by Elizabeth Casline and colleagues confirms that decreasing parental accommodation is vital to reducing child anxiety (Casline et al., 2018). Parental accommodation, defined as "changes in parents' behavior in attempts to prevent or reduce child distress," has been found to be strongly associated with generalized anxiety disorder, separation anxiety disorder, and specific phobias in children (Thompson-Hollands et al., 2014). Furthermore, when parents themselves suffer from an anxiety disorder, they may impart their cognitive styles to their children by influencing how they process their environment and emotions (Aktar et al., 2017). The child may learn that the world is not a safe place, strong emotions must be avoided, uncertainty cannot be tolerated, and worry is a coping strategy when faced with uncertainty.

In a 2019 review, Lisa-Marie Emerson and her colleagues investigated the role of parents in the development of child anxiety (Emerson et al., 2019). The reviewed studies affirm that parents contribute to their children's anxious cognitions via modeling fearful responses, which results in behavioral and emotional contagion. This limits their child's autonomy, as well as communicates their own expectations of their child's inability to cope with anxiety, thus further decreasing opportunities to practice independence. When a parent does not expect their child to be able to cope with a challenge, their child naturally comes to expect that they cannot cope with it either.

I hope it's become clear to you by now that I'm very non-judgmental of parents. I do not blame them for their child's mental health condition (except, of course, for abusive parents, whom I hold very accountable). Adolescent mental health problems exist within contexts and situations— temperamental influences, reinforcement patterns, unhelpful communication, as well as broader socio-cultural influences such as peer dynamics, expectation biases, helicopter parenting, and the effects of digital technology. When the circumstances and situations are positive and favorable, families and children thrive, and when they are not, serious problems can arise. All children and families are just trying to do the best they can from one day to the next, but they are generally unaware of the enormous role these influences are playing in their lives.

So, please do not take what I'm about to say as a criticism toward parents in any way. No judgment, it just is.

One of the ingredients that I see often with anxious-avoidant kids is a parental style that, while borne of love and affection, gets in the way of their child's well-being. Many of the anxious-avoidant kids that I've met have some of the most loving, committed, and attentive parents I've ever known. They are just good human beings in almost every respect. As I have mentioned before, any good quality to an extreme is no longer a good quality. It's obviously the job of all parents to protect their children, but, in many instances, the parents of anxious-avoidant children and teens are often so overly protective that it clearly works against the needs of the child and their mental health. Note too that over-protectiveness doesn't just affect kids who are avoidant; this same parental style can have exactly the same effect on depressed kids too.

So what does this look like? The expression I use with parents is "falling into the pool" with their child or teen. The parents have all the same age-appropriate expectations and want for their child—to engage fully in life and thrive—but these parents are much more susceptible to the "I can't do that" arguments made by the child. They come to believe these arguments— that the child isn't capable, that as parents they might be pushing too hard, that they could be making things worse, and that they are not being understanding enough. These parents are generally such kindhearted people that they back off really easily, and the child figures this out about them, much to the detriment of everyone in the family system.

Some of the saddest cases I have worked with involve parents who overprotect and have a hard time shifting away from this style into learning new behaviors that work much better. I can generally spot these parents early in treatment because, from the start, they resist the first, and generally the most benign, interventions I propose. In Chapter 3, I talked about the gentle-ask strategy, which entails starting with what I think of as "low-hanging fruit," some relatively small, easy-to-change behavior that usually comes toward the bottom of a problem hierarchy. I do this because I want an early win, to fix something small to get the child and their parents into a new rhythm of raising expectations, talking things through, and agreeing on some small ask, such as going to bed a little earlier or getting up to an alarm clock, or spending a little less time in their room. What happens with some overly protective parents, when the intervention is suggested, they are quick to try to talk me out of it by explaining why that's asking too much of the child. ("They need their phone at night to talk to their friends; otherwise, they're too anxious to sleep.") Almost always, after I present the rationale for the strategy, they will nod in agreement ... and then don't do it. To myself, I'm thinking, "If they're having trouble just asking their kid to go to bed a little earlier, just wait until we talk about the plan to get them to school every day." I do my very best to keep this very small subset of parents in treatment, but they often drop out after just a handful of sessions. Thankfully, most overprotective parents do, in fact, stay in treatment and are able to learn all the various strategies to vastly reduce their child's avoidant behavior.

The Role of Phones and Other Devices

As is often the case with children and adolescents with mental health issues, problematic use of phones and other devices plays a highly prominent role in the development and maintenance of anxious-avoidant behavior. In fact, I have almost never seen a family in which it hasn't played a role.

We learned previously, that there is a dose-related effect relative to device use—the longer a child or teen spends on a device (phone, tablet, etc.), the greater the risk of mental health problems. In my experience, most anxious-avoidant kids have few in-person friends, and so they turn to virtual communities to obtain a peer community. It is not at all uncommon for anxious teens to spend the vast majority of their time on a device. In most cases, parents intervene minimally—they generally do not set screen-time limits on their child's phone and don't do much monitoring of who they are communicating with and what is being said. Sometimes the parents don't know how to limit screen time, and/or they are afraid of how their child will react if they try to do so.

In addition to spending hours of unrestricted, unmonitored time each day on a device, many of the kids my colleagues and I work with have developed partial or even complete inverted sleep schedules—they stay up late at night and sleep in very late in the morning. As we have learned, devices greatly contribute to children and teens not getting enough sleep. Predictably, these kids are also very hard to wake up in the morning because of this, which leads to parents trying to wake them up over and over, setting the stage for a battle every day before school. When I hear of a child needing multiple prompts to wake up in the morning, coupled with morning irritability, my first (and usually correct) hypothesis is that they are up late on a device.

Excessive time on a device has additional side effects that we've previously discussed. It greatly de-incentivizes and often prevents kids from engaging in other, wellness-enhancing behaviors (the crowding out effect), such as spending time with family; getting exercise; being exposed to sunlight; and of course, ultimately, engaging in other age-typical behaviors and responsibilities. And, again, it's not just the amount of time on a device that causes problems, it's also important who the child is communicating with and about what. Almost all human beings have a need for connection, and so if a teen can't find this in real life, they are highly driven to find it virtually. As is the case with kids who self-harm, anxious-avoidant kids are also drawn to other teens and online communities that

182 Treating Social Isolation and Anxious Avoidance

are struggling with a similar mental health problem, setting the stage for emotional and behavioral contagion.

My observations of teenagers who participate in these online communities are that they are pretty well-versed in mental health and related topics. By versed, I don't mean knowledgeable, just that they spend a lot of time doing Google searches. We often have kids come to their parents and to us stating that they have this or that diagnosis based on their reading, and the more exotic the diagnosis the better. My best guess on this is that they are simply trying to find something, anything, that accounts for the state of their lives. It's along the lines of, "Well, no wonder I can't go to school or leave the house; I have x, y, and z." In the case of anxious-avoidant kids, doing the stuff of life can be difficult, so their motivation to latch onto a diagnosis as a causal explanation for their current inaction is understandable, but, of course, not at all helpful.

And there is another layer of complexity to all this as it relates to peers and virtual communities. In addition to echoing each other's avoidant and depressive feelings, it is my sense that kids in these communities often blame their parents for their own dysfunction. In a way this makes sense. Unfortunately, we live in a fairly blame-oriented society, so they certainly see blaming others modeled for them quite often. I see this blaming of parents in many instances of anxious avoidance (and with depressed and suicidal kids too but somewhat less often). I mentioned trauma earlier—this is common for kids to say—that they are the way they are because their parents have "traumatized" them. Trauma, of course, does lead to psychological problems, and in cases of physical, sexual, or emotional abuse, I'm right there with them.

However, in the majority of the families I have treated, while there have been hurts and upsets, I generally do not see anything in the family's history that meets the standards of trauma. Often when a kid is asked for specifics, the events they cite as proof of trauma just don't add up very well. In addition, they engage in a kind of reverse engineering based on their Google searches: "I can't function in life and I'm miserable. I learned I have borderline personality disorder (BPD) because I read about all of the symptoms. I also read that what leads to BPD is one or more traumatic experiences (sometimes but not always true of BPD), so therefore I must have been traumatized by something you did to me as a child that I may or may not be able to remember."

Before we move on to what to do about all of this, let's do a quick summary of what we know so far on the various situational and contextual factors that incentivize, promote, and maintain anxious-avoidant behavior.

It's important for both parents and the treating clinician to understand all of these influences so we don't bark up the wrong tree and spend our time focusing on (and trying to treat) the wrong things. We discussed the role of temperament, i.e., that some kids are just prone to be more anxious-leaning than other kids. The age-typical demands of adolescence are just going to be somewhat harder for them, and the principle of least effort tells us that avoidance does offer some advantages to kids in that it makes it possible for them to sometimes escape responsibilities that require sustained effort.

Reinforcement plays a significant role in anxious avoidance as well; if a task or responsibility is successfully avoided, the strategies implemented by the child to avoid those difficult tasks become reinforced, resulting in even more avoidant behavior. We learned that avoidant kids strongly resist their parents' attempts to re-engage them in life, and kids are often capable of creating guilt and doubt in their sometimes overprotective parents ("Why would you ask me to do things that make me even more anxious?").

In addition, devices play a key role in maintaining anxious-avoidant behaviors: The more time on a device, the greater the risk of worsening a child's mental health condition. It reduces opportunities for other well-being-enhancing activities, and additionally connects the child to virtual communities (echo chambers) that offer acceptance but also the encouragement of even more dysfunctional, avoidant behavior. Finally, as I mentioned earlier in the book, the overall cultural shift to helicopter parenting has decreased opportunities for kids to practice independence, which correlates with the increase in mental health challenges and a decrease in resilience among young people.

Now that we understand the situational variables that lead toward avoidant behavior, let's move on to treatment. And if you've learned anything about me at all up until now, you've probably already figured out that each of these factors must be disrupted or mitigated if we are going to draw a very reluctant teenager back out into the world.

Chief Takeaways from Chapter 9

For Parents

- You are the most powerful agents of change in your child's life—only you have the ability to change the situational variables that have promoted and now maintain your child's anxious-avoidant behavior. Therapists cannot do this.
- Be careful not to "fall into the pool," i.e., be talked out of asking your child to do hard things, or letting them convince you that you're asking too much of them.
- In order for your child to be less anxious and avoidant, they are going to need to engage in regular exposure activities, which they likely will not want to do.
- The only way kids become less afraid of something is by doing it over and over to the point at which they are no longer afraid.

For Clinicians

- Be prepared to encounter a lot of resistance from young patients when you start to encourage them to step back into life again.
- It is vital to perform a complete assessment of the various situational influences that are likely playing key roles in the development and maintenance of the child's avoidant behavior.
- Identify each of these influences and disrupt them one by one.
- Don't you "fall into the pool" either—kids will try to persuade you just as much as their parents. so that you don't ask things of them.
- When parents first start to ask their child or teenager to engage in life more, it's going to be a scary time for them. They likely have an overprotective style that comes from a place of deep love and affection, so they'll need lots of support and encouragement when you start asking them to do things differently.

References

Abramowitz, J. S., Deacon, B. J., & Whiteside, S. P. H. (2011). *Exposure therapy for anxiety: Principles and practice* (2nd ed.). Guilford Press.

Aktar, E., Nikolić, M., & Bögels, S. M. (2017). Environmental transmission of generalized anxiety disorder from parents to children: Worries, experiential avoidance, and intolerance of uncertainty. *Dialogues in Clinical Neuroscience, 19*(2), 137–147. 10.31887/DCNS.2017.19.2/eaktar

Albano, A. M. (2020, May 27). *How to raise kids who can overcome anxiety* [Video]. TED Conferences. https://www.ted.com/talks/anne_marie_albano_how_to_raise_kids_who_can_overcome_anxiety

American Academy of Child and Adolescent Psychiatry. (n.d.). *Your adolescent - anxiety and avoidant disorders.* https://www.aacap.org/aacap/Families_and_Youth/Resource_Centers/Anxiety_Disorder_Resource_Center/Your_Adolescent_Anxiety_and_Avoidant_Disorders.aspx

American Psychological Association. (2017, July). *What is exposure therapy?* https://www.apa.org/ptsd-guideline/patients-and-families/exposure-therapy

Bennett, E. D., Le, K., Lindahl, K., Wharton, S., & Mak, T. W. (2017). *Five out of the box techniques for encouraging teenagers to engage in counseling.* American Counseling Association. https://www.counseling.org/docs/default-source/vistas/encouraging-teenagers.pdf

Bertelsen, T. B., Wergeland, G. J., Nordgreen, T., Himle, J. A., & Haland, A. T. (2022). Benchmarked effectiveness of family and school involvement in group exposure therapy for adolescent anxiety disorder. *Psychiatry Research, 313,* Article 114632. 10.1016/j.psychres.2022.114632

Casline, E. P., Pella, J., Zheng, D., Harel, O., Drake, K. L., & Ginsburg, G. S. (2018). Parental responses to children's avoidance in fear-provoking situations: Relation to child anxiety and mediators of intervention response. *Child & Youth Care Forum*, 47, 443–462. 10.1007/s10566-018-9440-7

Emerson, L.-M., Ogielda, C., & Rowse, G. (2019). A systematic review of the role of parents in the development of anxious cognitions in children. *Journal of Anxiety Disorders*, 62, 15–25. 10.1016/j.janxdis.2018.11.002

Foa, E. B., & Andrews, L. W. (2006). *If your adolescent has an anxiety disorder: An essential resource for parents.* Oxford University Press.

Hawes, M., Szenczy, A., Klein, D., Hajcak, G., & Nelson, B. (2022). Increases in depression and anxiety symptoms in adolescents and young adults during the COVID-19 pandemic. *Psychological Medicine*, 52(14), 3222–3230. 10.1017/S0033291720005358

Holly, E., & Pina, A. (2015). Variations in the influence of parental socialization of anxiety among clinic referred children. *Child Psychiatry & Human Development*, 46(3), 474–484. 10.1007/s10578-014-0487-x

Kremer, W., & Hammond, C. (2013, July 5). Hikikomori: Why are so many Japanese men refusing to leave their rooms? *BBC News.* https://www.bbc.com/news/magazine-23182523

Landro, L. (2013, May 27). A better way to treat anxiety. *The Wall Street Journal.* https://www.wsj.com/articles/SB10001424127887323475304578503584007049700

Lorenzo, N. E., Zeytinoglu, S., Morales, S., Listokin, J., Almas, A. N., Degnan, K. A., Henderson, H., Chronis-Tuscano, A., & Fox, N. A. (2021). Transactional associations between parent and late adolescent internalizing symptoms during the COVID-19 pandemic: The moderating role of avoidant coping. *Journal of Youth and Adolescence*, 50, 459–469. 10.1007/s10964-020-01374-z

National Institute of Mental Health. (n.d.). *Anxiety disorders.* U.S. Department of Health and Human Services, National Institutes of Health. https://www.nimh.nih.gov/health/topics/anxiety-disorders

Peris, T. S., Storch, E. A., & McGuire, J. (Eds.). (2020). *Exposure therapy for children with anxiety and OCD: Clinician's guide to integrated treatment.* Academic Press.

Racine, N., McArthur, B. A., Cooke, J. E., Eirich, R., Zhu, J., & Madigan, S. (2021). Global prevalence of depressive and anxiety symptoms in children and adolescents during COVID-19: A meta-analysis. *JAMA Pediatrics*, 175(11), 1142–1150. 10.1001/jamapediatrics.2021.2482

Southam-Gerow, M. A. (2019). *Exposure therapy with children and adolescents.* The Guilford Press.

Teunisse, A. K., Pembroke, L., O'Gradey-Lee, M., Sy, M., Rapee, R. M., Wuthrich, V. M., Creswell, C., & Hudson, J. L. (2022). A scoping review investigating the use of exposure for the treatment and targeted prevention of anxiety and related disorders in young people. *JCPP Advances*, 2(2), Article e12080. 10.1002/jcv2.12080

Thompson-Hollands, J., Kerns, C. E., Pincus, D. B., & Comer, J. S. (2014). Parental accommodation of child anxiety and related symptoms: Range, impact, and correlates. *Journal of Anxiety Disorders*, 28(8), 765–773. 10.1016/j.janxdis.2014.09.007

Tice, A. M. B. (2019). Adapting an exposure and response prevention manual to treat youth obsessive-compulsive disorder and comorbid anxiety disorder: The case of "Daniel." *Pragmatic Case Studies in Psychotherapy*, *15*(1), 1–74. 10.14713/pcsp.v15i1.2043

Wang, S., Chen, L., Ran, H., Che, Y., Fang, D., Sun, H., Peng, J., Liang, X., & Xiao, Y. (2022). Depression and anxiety among children and adolescents pre and post COVID-19: A comparative meta-analysis. *Frontiers in Psychiatry*, *13*, Article 917552. 10.3389/fpsyt.2022.917552

Whiteside, S. P. H., Ollendick, T. H., & Biggs, B. K. (2020). *Exposure therapy for child and adolescent anxiety and OCD*. Oxford University Press.

10 The Treatment of Anxious Avoidance from a Family-Focused Perspective

We have now laid the foundation for how kids like Lucas, described in Chapter 9, end up becoming so completely fearful and avoidant of most of the age-typical activities and responsibilities of adolescent life. We've learned that they are the product of the various temperamental and situational influences that created and currently maintain the avoidant behaviors. However, let's turn our attention to disrupting these influences so highly avoidant children and adolescents can be far less anxious and much more engaged in life.

The Role of Parents

The anxious, avoidant child or teen needs their parents' help desperately, probably more than any other group of patients with whom I work. They simply cannot pull themselves out of their avoidant pattern without the sustained effort and support from their families. I also strongly believe that the last thing these kids need is to be sent to an individual therapist who does not include family in their treatment. Many of the anxious-avoidant patients that we treat have already had quite a bit of individual therapy, often for years, but with no perceivable improvement of any kind. The reason for this seems obvious. No therapist working with just the child or teen has anywhere near the kind of power or influence necessary to effect meaningful change to address the situational variables that resulted in the child's current avoidant behavior.

How can an individual therapist disrupt an over-protective (enabling) parental style without ever meeting with the parents? And what about doing the exposure therapy itself? An individual therapist working alone can spend considerable time talking with a child or adolescent about the value of exposure therapy, but unless they are willing to go to the child's house and take them on a driving lesson or be with them while they drop off job applications, the conversations alone will be of little value.

DOI: 10.4324/9781003397366-14

Any successful form of treatment must be focused on helping the child's parents approach the problem in a very different way. Change in the system begins with them because they are the only ones who have enough power and influence to change the situational variables that are negatively influencing the child or teen's behavior. A therapist might not be able to be with the child or teen as they do exposure work, but parents certainly can. As we learned in Chapter 7, parents play a significant role in the treatment of suicidal and self-harming behavior, but this is especially true in the treatment of anxious avoidance.

Key Parent Behaviors to Target for Change

Creating an Environment of Optimism and Expectation

I believe it is imperative that the very first thing that needs to happen in families with an anxious-avoidant child is to create an entirely new climate of expectation: "We believe you can do this and you must." For so long, in some cases for years, the bar for the child in the family has gradually been lowered to the point where the patient has adopted the belief that they are somehow damaged goods, and in many ways, they are simply acting out that lowered expectation.

It would be difficult for the kid to believe otherwise. They are fully aware of the fact that their life in no way resembles that of a normal teenager—far from it. Living in fear of everyday experiences, having few or no friends, no aspirations or an expectation of a life that's big enough to be worth living; being stuck in their bedroom, and only interacting with the world virtually is not a recipe for a child to feel good about themselves. These kids are miserable without exception. They absolutely know that they are in a bad situation but have no idea how they got there, much less what to do to get out, or even where to start.

In addition, if you were to ask them what their preference is—to get started now facing up to their fears or to wait until they are feeling better to do so, every one of them will say they want to wait (avoid longer). I find there is a general belief among therapists, at least as it applies to children, that is often fundamentally wrong: Work with the client so that they can feel better and then they will start doing better.

Perhaps this is true in some cases, but with most children and teens, it is actually the reverse: Once kids start doing better, they feel better. I have seen this borne out over and over in my work, i.e., when we create new situational variables that directly result in positive behavioral change, these kids thrive. They look better, sound better, and report feeling better simply because we carefully and strategically engineered the environment in such a way that resulted in them behaving in a different, more positive, and functional way.

Parents need a tremendous amount of support and therapeutic guidance to pull this off. It requires that they let go of old habits that don't work and replace them with strategies that do. Changing well-entrenched patterns of behavior at home comes only with the parents' effort and willingness to put their child in challenging situations.

It is very important for parents to communicate their optimism to their child with respect to change and to be relentless in their pursuit of it. It is here that shifts in language can be very effective. Rather than having long, extended conversations with their teen in which they try to persuade them to do something they are disinclined to do, it is far more effective for parents to let go of persuading and slip into the role of gently, but firmly, requiring. For example, if a child or teen says, "I'm too anxious to go to school today," rather than trying to persuade them of the value of school, it is far more effective to say in a matter-of-fact way, "I know some days are harder than others, but school is important. I'm confident you can go, even if it's hard." The words, of course, need to match the parents' body language and facial expressions. You can't just say the words; words must be backed up by a tone and presentation that comes across as upbeat and confident. In doing so, the parent capitalizes on what we know about emotional contagion: Optimism spreads.

Most parents, in my experience, spend far too much time trying to talk their anxious-avoidant child into doing things they are not keen to do. It makes sense that this would happen in families. After all, this is what adults do with each other. How else do we persuade another adult to do something other than pointing out the value of doing so? However, as I have talked about before, kids don't necessarily think like adults or respond to the same strategy an adult might. There should be a little persuasion, of course, but more than a little usually results in an unnecessary tug-of-war, which only gives the child incentive to dig in further and throw more counterarguments at the parent.

In truth, it can be very hard to persuade someone of something when they are operating under powerful incentives not to believe it. Remember the avoidant child is driven by fear. Their incentive not to buy their parents' arguments about the value of doing hard things is motivated by this, hence persuasion will in most cases be ineffective. The solution is to stop trying to persuade and instead gently, confidently, but firmly, insist.

An example of communicating confidence and expectation is when a child texts repeatedly from school asking to be picked up. They often call or text repeatedly, citing the many reasons why they can't stay in school, most of which will probably sound very familiar to parents:

"I'm too anxious to be here today."
"I just can't handle it anymore."

"Something just happened and you have to come pick me up."
"My teacher embarrassed me so I can't finish the day."
"Another kid was being mean and so I'm so stressed that I left class."
"I promise if you come get me I'll go back tomorrow."

In this type of situation, we first coach parents to be very slow in their response to the text. Sending an immediate response creates the impression that the situation is urgent when in truth it really is not. Anxiety is uncomfortable but it is not an emergency. Depending on the situation, responding in a leisurely 30 to 60 minutes sends this important message, with each subsequent text similarly spaced out. Being slow to respond gives the child an opportunity to successfully navigate whatever the problem is on their own, thus instilling a sense of mastery and competence.

The second piece of coaching we provide is that parents should never respond to the details of the child's argument or get pulled into a back-and-forth about the source of their anxiety. Doing so makes it too easy to "fall into the pool" and become convinced by the child that they should be picked up. Far better parent responses are those that are neutral but communicate confidence and the clear expectation that the child can successfully tolerate their anxiety and get through it, such as: "That sounds challenging but I'm sure you'll make it work" or "I'm sorry someone said something unkind. That's no fun. Let me know when you're back in class."

Enabling Parents to Stop Enabling

If we can reasonably surmise that there is an element of enabling that takes place in these families, then the clinician must take steps to disrupt this unhelpful pattern. The first step in helping parents to stop rescuing and enabling their child is for them to understand and agree with the rationale for doing so. If parents don't understand the reason for changing their behavior they simply won't. This is a very difficult part of treatment, which requires quite a lot of clinical attention. It begins with psychoeducation: Here's what we know about how anxiety disorders develop; the various ways avoidance serves to keep the anxiety alive over time; that treatment entails opposite action (the child facing the thing that scares them often enough so that it no longer scares them); how not insisting that your child do hard things is a big part of the problem; and why it's infinitely better for the child to start on this now rather than waiting until they say they're ready to start (which, again, practically never happens).

For parents to shift their own behavior is, in many cases, quite challenging. Rescuing or enabling parental behavior ultimately comes from a good place, i.e., a desire on the parents' part to love and protect their child. It's every parent's instinct to want their child to feel better, and to step in and quickly relieve their child's distress. Often in treatment, the rationale for giving the child or teen opportunities to face challenges on their own must be revisited many times by the therapist, lest the parents slip back into old habits of enabling.

This unhelpful pattern of reinforcement (the child avoiding and then the parents backing down), must be disrupted by the clinician. In the example of the child calling from school asking to be picked up, the parent has to stand firm on their position: "I won't pick you up when you call me from school. I'd be sending you the wrong message if I did and in a way, I'd be agreeing with you that it's not possible to stay in class. I'm confident that you can do hard things, including this. I know that's not what you want but I'm doing it anyway."

The Treatment Hierarchy and Gentle Ask

In IFFT, at the start of treatment, we collaborate with the parents to develop a treatment and exposure hierarchy, a wish list so to speak, of where in the child's life avoidance is currently taking place and the specific behaviors that we're going to focus our efforts on changing. We often try to collaborate with the child on this as well and some of them may be willing to participate in developing the plan. However, we find most severely anxious and avoidant kids are highly resistant to the idea of change and often to treatment in general. (We'll talk shortly about resistance and what to do about it.)

The wish list is arranged from what we suspect will be the least challenging behavior for the child to tackle up to what is very likely going to be the most challenging. We always start with the easiest behavior on the list, the one most amenable to change, and work our way up from there. We simply can't tackle everything all at once, and if we were to attempt to do so we would stress the family system too quickly and overwhelm both the parents and the child.

For example, the following might be a potential wish list, arranged in a treatment hierarchy, from what we suspect will be least challenging for the child to change to the most challenging:

Cleaning their bedroom
Spending less time in their bedroom and more time with family (even for very brief periods)
Helping out around the house by doing chores
Spending less time at home: going on a walk with family, out for lunch, a short trip somewhere, a visit to extended family, and so on
Showering and brushing their teeth daily

If the child is not in school, engaging in some type of online learning
  daily
Completing homework
Going to school in person

If the teen is old enough, completing the steps necessary to get their driver's license and a part-time job *[Side note: we always advocate for kids doing chores, getting their license, and getting a part-time job. We do this because it is consistent with the research indicating these tasks in particular contribute to the development of independence and resiliency. These activities are just a part of growing up as well.]*

We will always employ the gentle-ask strategy with each one of these in turn as we progress through treatment. Again, this entails simply asking the child, either in a family therapy session or at home, to consider doing something different. It's worded something like this: "Hey you hang out in your room quite a bit. We miss seeing you and wonder what you'd think about joining us for a family movie night once a week?" Most kids will say yes to this, but if they say they can't (or won't) for whatever reason, a good reply to that is: "Well, we'd love it if you tried." Agreeing to the request, of course, doesn't mean they'll actually do it, but a fair number of kids finally will do it if their parents stay persistent and friendly. If that doesn't work, we will revisit the ask each week for several weeks, and if that still doesn't work we will look for ways to leverage incentives, usually access to devices (more on this in just a bit).

Parent Therapy Sessions

In IFFT, the vast majority of the work to change how the parents respond to their child's avoidance takes place in the parent sessions. Most of the focus over the course of treatment is on encouraging parents to remain steady in their pursuit of change and providing enough guidance and support to maintain positive momentum when things become challenging. And it most definitely will become challenging. In most cases when the parents start to move away from enabling and rescuing behavior, kids who have become accustomed to it will often double down on trying to convince their parents that they're doing the wrong thing ("How can you ask me to do this? You're making my anxiety worse. Is that what you want?"). From the child's perspective, this makes sense—they are no longer receiving reinforcement for talking their way out of things, so their natural response is to try even harder to talk their way out of things.

When a parent begins to shift their own behavior and stops reinforcing their child's avoidance and also raises their expectations that the child start doing difficult things, this creates an upset in the family's equilibrium. The child or teen is being temporarily stressed, which, in turn, causes stress on the parents. To get through this difficult phase in treatment, most parents need ongoing reassurance that they are doing the right thing, even if their child tries to convince them otherwise. The parents' therapist also needs to be vigilant and address any instances in which the parents are tempted to swoop in and rescue the child from their distress. I find this happens quite a bit throughout the treatment process so it's really important to keep an eye out for it.

The path out of all this is a difficult one for both the parents and the child, but once some initial success is achieved, parents start to gradually become more and more confident in their new abilities. As this occurs, they also witness progress in both the child's behavior and how the child feels, creating a positive feedback loop that accelerates the child's ability to take on newer, more challenging exposure tasks.

Family Therapy Sessions

For the anxious-avoidant child, family therapy sessions are focused on discussions aimed at facilitating the exposure process and reducing conflict that arises when the child becomes resistant. Young patients will often use family therapy as a forum to talk their parents out of asking more of them. The therapist is present to facilitate a dialog between family members to help them learn each other's perspectives, but this does not mean that the entire hour is filled with giving the teen a platform to tell their parents they are doing the wrong thing. Similar to the advice given in the parent session, the therapist is there to model and teach everyone how to better communicate with each other, but not allow a protracted debate that goes nowhere. Once the therapist has judged that sufficient time has been devoted to the topic, they will close that part of the discussion by saying something like, "Well, it sounds like your parents are pretty set on your taking a shower every day. I know that's not what you want but everyone now has had time to voice their concerns. Let's move on to a different topic of conversation."

Individual and Skills Training Sessions

As parents become better at asking for and holding higher expectations for the child, a great deal of additional therapeutic work takes place in the individual and skills training sessions. Once the therapist and the child have formed a good relationship, in many cases, kids are far more open to having conversations with them about the value of change than they are with their parents. I think that's because therapists aren't, well, parental. Therapists never tell kids what to do. Instead, we influence kids' perspectives on things through a combination of warmth, humor, persistence, offering advice, and the various other tricks of our trade. For example, if using a DBT or CBT perspective, a therapist can gently challenge and restructure any negative beliefs that might be fueling the avoidance. If the current belief is "I can't go to school because kids make fun of me," the therapist can help identify any distortions in that thought (in this case fortune telling and catastrophizing) and help the child or teen replace that belief with: "It's possible some kids might make fun of me but not necessarily, and even if they do I know how to handle it." Kids tend to be more receptive to this type of help from someone other than their parents, even if their parents were to say exactly the same thing to them.

In the skills training sessions, typically the approach would be heavily oriented toward teaching the child various different DBT techniques and strategies to cope better with anxiety. This might include deep breathing, some type of distraction technique, visualization, and the like. Some anxious-avoidant kids make great use of DBT skills, but in my experience, many do not, especially when they are still at the resistance stage and of the mindset that they are not capable of doing difficult things. For kids who won't use skills, either because they are stubborn or for any other reason, the therapist reminds them that just learning to tolerate their distress is a viable alternative, and they express confidence that the child can learn to do so.

Resistance and Leveraging New Behavior

Avoidant children and teens, especially those who are as incapacitated as Lucas in the vignette, are often some of the most resistant kids I see in my practice, and understandably so.

I think what happens to people—children and adults—when they avoid anxiety-inducing situations for long periods of time (often years, in the case of many of my patients), it becomes increasingly difficult to return to those situations. Many of us experienced that same phenomenon with the pandemic—the shelter-at-home orders effectively prevented most of the typical social encounters to which we are accustomed. In my case, once the restrictions started to lift, I just felt rusty when it came to interacting with others. I still remembered how to do it, obviously, but I just felt off somehow until my life as usual fully resumed and I was back in the swing of things. Additionally, for me, after the pandemic was over, I essentially stepped right back into the world with which I was very familiar.

We know that the pandemic has worsened the mental health of many kids, so I'm sure an element of this is coming into play. Couple that with an anxious temperament, especially with kids who are a bit socially awkward on top of that. Also imagine a teenager out of school possibly for years, spending most of their time isolated in their bedroom—think how much their social world has changed around them during this time period. Adolescence is like a fast-moving river. If a kid steps out of it, even for a brief period of time, how can they not feel like the world has left them behind?

Would I be anxious and avoidant in that same situation? Absolutely I would. Would I be highly resistant when someone asks that I do the opposite of my inclination and do really hard, scary things? Absolutely.

It's just not a surprise, therefore, that many highly avoidant kids who enter treatment are highly resistant to change. We know that persuading them to engage in challenging situations doesn't work. Goodness knows, their parents have tried this for years with no success. Well, what about therapists then? Maybe they can get them to try harder things. Sometimes, yes, but in many cases, no, again because we don't have the power to alter negative situational variables.

The gentle ask does work sometimes. If the parents and the kid's therapist are persistent, there are some patients who will, in fact, spend less time in their rooms or occasionally leave the house. However, for kids like Lucas, the gentle ask, even if coupled with all of the skills employed by the therapist, simply does not work and the child or teen remains mostly, or even exclusively, avoidant and will sit out that fast-moving river and never jump back in. Life will pass them by, year after year, which is why we've all known at least one family with an unmotivated adult still living at home paralyzed by life, utterly despondent, and feeling miserable about themselves and the world in general.

If after working for several weeks with a family, trying the various different strategies described in this chapter thus far, the child continues to refuse to engage even in the least challenging behavior on the hierarchy (or gets stuck somewhere higher up on the hierarchy), it's time to shift gears and incentivize them.

In terms of incentives, we start by looking at what privileges the child or teen has now and try to identify those that we can leverage to our (and ultimately the child's) advantage. By incentives, I am not referring to offering rewards or contracts because in my experience these do not have sufficient power to motivate kids to overcome their avoidance.

However, there is one option that is almost always available—access to their devices. I have never once, not ever, met a highly anxious and avoidant kid who didn't spend hours and hours each day on their phone or other device. It makes sense that they would, because like all kids, avoidant kids also want some kind of social connection, and a device is a gateway to the world, even if accessed in a passive way. And just from a practical perspective, they need some way to pass an entire day, and phones are designed to keep us and our kids engaged for long periods of time. Limiting screen time is an important part of treatment for all of our IFFT patients for the many reasons described throughout this book, so leveraging devices to give kids incentive to take on new challenges fits into this nicely as well.

Here is what that looks like. Again, we don't start by leveraging devices, we begin with the gentle ask and accompanying efforts by the individual and skills training therapists and stick with that for several weeks. In family therapy, the parents keep revisiting the ask (to maybe come out of their room more often, help out around the house, and so on) each week in session, with the support of the therapist. It's possible the child keeps agreeing to the ask but still isn't doing it, or perhaps they steadfastly refuse to do it altogether. In either case, eventually, the time comes to leverage and the conversation sounds something like this:

Parent (P): So, we've talked for a while now about you helping out around the house, maybe doing one chore a day, yeah?

Child (C): Yeah.

P: Well, what's going on with that?

C: I said I would do it.

P: It's true but you haven't.

C: Why can't I do it when I'm ready? I don't understand why you're pushing me. That makes me even more anxious.

P: Well, I don't mean to make you anxious, but it's important that you help out around the house even so.

C: I will when I'm feeling better. Why can't you understand this? I think you should learn more about how anxiety works so you can stop making so many mistakes.

P: I know this is new for you, but we're going to ask you to start doing one chore a day even if it makes you anxious. We're pretty confident you can make that work.

C: No, I can't make that work and I don't want to talk about this anymore.

P: Well, here's the thing. You'll probably disagree, but we think your phone is playing a part in this problem, given how much time you spend on it. How about each day we start with your phone turned off? Happy to turn it back on after you've done your chore? Seem fair?

C: So the ONE THING that makes me feel better you're going to take away from me? How does that help me? I'm not letting you turn my phone off. That's not happening.

P: Tell you what, we'll give you a couple of days to start doing your chore, and that way you can keep your phone. But, come the end of the week, if you're still not doing it by then, we'll turn off your phone until the chore is done. This starts tomorrow.

C: I don't know why you're punishing me! I'm keeping my phone and I'm not doing your stupid chores!

P: Do your chores or not, that's up to you, just understand what the consequence is for not doing them. But, we're not going to argue or debate it with you.

Kids absolutely hate it when parents first start doing this. Of course, they will try to argue or debate it endlessly, but we teach parents how to end the conversation and just walk away if they need to. Sometimes the threat alone of taking their phones is enough to elicit the new behavior, but most of the time not. Parents have to make good on taking the phone and hold their ground as the child protests. We often have to teach parents how to disable devices remotely because many kids will not hand them over willingly, but there are many effective ways to do this. In my experience, over the course of a few weeks, the protests will gradually taper off into fairly age-typical grumbling, and after a month or two the teen will be in the habit of doing chores quite successfully. Parents are often very shocked (and pleased) to see their child or teen do their chores when, just a few weeks before, the kid insisted they couldn't do them.

Leveraging devices in this manner is almost always highly effective, even for the most avoidant (and oppositional) kids. In fact, I've not seen an occasion in which it wasn't effective. We will use this same strategy as we work our way up the treatment hierarchy, all the way to the top. For example, if we're on the last step and say we're now working on the teen getting a job, the parent will employ the same strategy ("Happy to turn your phone back on after you've submitted three job applications online each day."). Ultimately, I believe kids know they need help moving forward and want to do so. Leveraging their devices is a way for them to get over their inertia, and it likely provides a face-saving way for them to do so ("My parents made me come back to school."). Again, as I've mentioned before, once kids actually start to re-engage in life and begin to learn they truly can do hard things, their self-esteem improves dramatically and they give every indication of being far happier kids.

I spoke earlier of how the family system will become stressed, especially early on in treatment, as the parents shift away from enabling and rescuing to increasing their expectations of the child or teen. Leveraging devices adds an additional layer of stress, so the importance of doing this safely cannot be overstated. If you are a parent reading this, do not attempt this on your own. An experienced, highly skilled therapist is essential if this strategy is employed, and only then after a careful safety assessment. This is especially true if the avoidant patient also engages in self-harming behavior (not uncommon for avoidance and self-harm to go together), and in this case, even more clinical skill is needed as safety is paramount. Of course, no parent should attempt to use this strategy without professional help.

Let's now turn our attention to Lucas, the kid in the previous chapter, and find out what becomes of him.

Chief Takeaways from Chapter 10

For Parents

- In order to best help your child, a good first step is to ask yourself whether you sometimes come to their rescue when they are faced with something challenging. It is really important to let kids solve their own problems when appropriate, and sometimes that means learning from failure too.
- Attempts at persuasion usually just lead to frustration and give your child or teen an incentive to come up with even better arguments as to why they should keep avoiding.
- Know that your child or teen doesn't want to be this way and is relying on you to help them in ways that will be difficult for you, at least initially.
- Kids feel better once they start doing better, not the other way around. Start with the doing and the positive feelings will come after.
- Assume your child or teen is capable, rather than assuming they can't do something. Set the bar high and don't be afraid to ask your kids to do hard things, because that's what builds confidence and resiliency.

For Clinicians

- If you alone are treating a highly avoidant and resistant patient without involving their parents, you are probably doing the child and the family a disservice unless you are making clear, unequivocal progress.
- Start to effect change by targeting the "low-hanging fruit," the first item on the exposure hierarchy. This will build up the parents' confidence that their child is capable of doing hard things.
- Let go of persuasion yourself—some attempts at this are okay and even helpful at times, but, like parents, you'll very likely need to be far more focused on incentivizing the child and supporting efforts at doing so.
- Don't be afraid to encourage parents to use the most powerful incentive available: Their child or teen's devices. In my experience, this almost always has more than sufficient power to bring about enormous improvement in the child's behavior.
- Optimism spreads. Believe in a family's ability to change, and they will too.

11 Case Example of Treating Anxious Avoidance

The Boy Who Disappeared

This is the second of our two case examples, and, as I did in the first, I have masked the identifying information of this patient and his family to protect their privacy. In every other respect, however, the details of what unfolded in the patient's treatment are just as they occurred. The case of Lucas is a reasonably good representation of the severely anxious and avoidant patients that my colleagues and I treat. His case was a bit harder than most, as we shall see, but his story contains many of the key elements that make avoidant kids so challenging for parents and clinicians.

"Lucas" was 17 years old when his parents first contacted our clinic to see if he was a candidate for IFFT. While always a shy and somewhat anxious kid, Lucas's life and development were fairly normal until about four years before. During that time period, Lucas came out as a transgender male (he was assigned female at birth), but it didn't appear as if that played any significant role in what was going on. However, I'll talk a bit more about this shortly. I suspect the start of Lucas's decline coincided with him getting his first laptop, and like many young people, he began to spend increasing amounts of time online isolated in his bedroom, and less and less time interacting with his two parents and the outside world.

I adored his parents. I have genuinely liked almost all of the parents with whom I've come into contact over the years, but this was especially true of them. They were both just the nicest, gentlest of human beings. Lucas's mother worked for a nonprofit organization and his father was a chemist. Their love for their child was abundant, and they would clearly go to the ends of the earth for him. Lucas's parents were, however, at their wit's end, and understandably so. I used the metaphor of the frog in the pot of water in Chapter 9, and this captures their experience perfectly. It was not any one thing that they could put their finger on, just a slow, gradual change from a completely functional middle-school kid to someone anything but that.

Lucas's parents did initially regulate his time on his laptop. He would have time limits on it, and they made sure he'd also do other things each

DOI: 10.4324/9781003397366-15

day, but they gradually let go of regulating his time on it. Some of it was probably just assuming whatever Lucas was doing online was harmless (as many parents do), and he seemed content enough at first. Gradually, however, any in-person friendships Lucas had were falling by the wayside and he began to connect with others only virtually. He would not talk about any of these people, except to say that he communicated with them on Discord.

I can't say that I'm an expert on Discord, but through my work with teenagers and young adults, I've been able to glean some useful information. What started out as a platform for gamers to communicate with each other seems to have morphed into a much larger and broader community for adolescents and young adults. More accurately, it's comprised of sub-communities, which function like chat rooms that are theme- or topic-oriented. While I am certain that Discord brings together many like-minded teens in helpful and positive ways, it also appears to me (or at least at the time of this writing) to often be a refuge for disaffected, unhappy young people. Many of the teens and young adults I treat who are struggling with depression and anxiety gravitate to Discord. When they tell me about who they are communicating with on the platform, many of the kids in these sub-communities seem equally depressed and anxious. It raises the concern again of echo chambers, i.e., a mutual reinforcement of dysfunction via social contagion. If the only people that a depressed and anxious young person talks to are also depressed and anxious, logic tells you this is not likely to be a helpful influence in a child's life. In my practice, I recommend to parents that they monitor their child's activity on Discord, especially if the child has a serious mental health condition with few or no in-person friends. Therapists could help their patients as well by asking them about their experiences on Discord and assessing what effects, if any, these experiences might be having on their well-being.

I have no evidence other than anecdotal to back this up, but it appears to me that part of the discussions that take place on Discord (and other platforms too, I'm sure), seems to include an element of blaming parents. I think when one's life has not turned out to be the way we had hoped, there is a natural human tendency to want to point the finger at someone. In truth, their unhappiness in life often isn't their parents' fault, or anyone else's for that matter. The fault lies in the teen's current circumstances and situational influences, and until those are disrupted and replaced by more favorable ones, they will continue to be miserable.

I had a young adult patient once and he and I would have many conversations about his experiences with his friends he met Discord. He was an anxious-avoidant person too, frozen in life, and living at home with his parents. His mood was predominantly low, not because he had a "mood disorder," but because he had what would be best characterized as a life circumstances disorder. His relationship with his family wasn't great for a number of reasons beyond his control, and he was only minimally employed doing work from home. Like the rest of us, though, he wanted social connections. Developing a community of friendships via Discord worked well for him (although this perpetuated his avoidance to some degree), so consequently I had the opportunity to observe his social world over several years. The people he connected with on Discord were by and large in the same situation as him: Depressed and avoidant; not working; spending most of their time on a device; having only virtual relationships; and hating and rarely speaking to their parents. My patient was in an echo chamber, clearly, and it was doing him no favors.

This same patient was very intelligent and mature for his age (actually more mature than many adults I have met), but these traits worked against him when it came to his online relationships. It seemed as if just about everyone he connected with on Discord was anything but mature. It was clear that their social skills and ability to navigate interpersonal relationships needed quite a bit of work (to say the least), so eventually each friendship unraveled one by one through no fault of his own. Eventually, he was left with no healthy online relationships, so this motivated him to cultivate in-person friendships with people who, thankfully, were more mature and interpersonally skilled, not anxious or depressed, and employed in work beyond minimum-wage jobs. My patient's mood steadily improved and his anxiety lessened simply because he managed to pull himself out of that dysfunctional echo chamber. (He also got a job that led to a meaningful career, which made an enormous difference as well.)

Lucas was angry at his parents too. He would often comment that he was upset with them because when he first came out as trans, they were not supportive and therefore transphobic. That struck me as odd because in none of my interactions with his parents did I see any indication of that. They were, in fact, very progressive and didn't seem to have any issues with Lucas transitioning at all. I've seen the opposite of this many times in my practice and I know what transphobic looks like. When asked in what ways specifically his parents were not supportive of his transitioning, Lucas responded with vague statements such as: "Well, it took them a long time to use the correct pronoun." Okay, that's fair enough I suppose, but when asked how long it took them to start using the "he" pronoun consistently, Lucas said, "I don't know, at least a few weeks." I am absolutely certain that Lucas was communicating online with other trans kids who had horror stories of their own coming-out experience, so it's not a stretch to wonder if Lucas had absorbed some of these stories and woven them into his own personal narrative to the point where he believed them to be true. I think Lucas was stuck in a life that was in no way "normal," and as many kids with mental health challenges do, he looked for ways to make sense of that by looking outside of himself.

Discord or not, Lucas's laptop very likely was a key ingredient in the onset of his anxious avoidance. Once his parents started to suspect this as well, they tried to limit his time on it, but it did not go well at all. As one might expect, Lucas became very argumentative, which gradually progressed into his becoming explosive. As we discussed earlier, Lucas's parents fell into the habit of giving in to him to reduce conflict, thereby reinforcing his behavior each time he argued. When they would muster the courage to be firm, it only gave him incentive to argue even more (and come up with arguments that were increasingly persuasive). He finally learned, as many kids do, that if he just got mad or belligerent, his parents would acquiesce, as they had become afraid of him and what he might do. Lucas does not have an "anger management problem" as we so often hear. Rather, his angry behavior was learned, and because his parents inadvertently reinforced it many times, the function of his anger (the purpose it served) was to ensure he could remain on his laptop. Again, there is no judgment here toward Lucas—this is just what happens when parents inadvertently reinforce the wrong thing.

In addition to spending most of his time online and isolated in his bedroom, Lucas began to report more and more depression and anxiety, which eventually led to additional avoidant behavior. He went to school less and less often, eventually refusing to go altogether. His parents asked for and received an assessment for special education services, and Lucas qualified under what is referred to in the U.S. as "emotionally disturbed," an awful name that, shockingly, no one has ever changed. (Actually, it used to be called "seriously emotionally disturbed," which is such a small improvement that I am not sure why they even bothered with it at all.) Lucas's school placed him on an independent study program at home, but he refused to do any work or meet with the teacher who was sent to his house ("I'm too anxious to meet with her"). His school pretty much left it at that, and at the time our services began, Lucas had no viable way of graduating from high school.

Lucas gradually began to refuse to do anything else, in each case citing his anxiety. He would not do any chores around the house, or even small tasks like carrying in the groceries when his mother came back from the store. If her hands were full and she rang the bell to be let in, Lucas would just stay on his bed and ignore her. He almost never left the house to run errands or take trips or vacations with his family. Hygiene was a significant problem as well. His parents reported that he had only bathed or brushed his teeth a handful of times in the previous four years.

Despite all the various problems that Lucas was struggling with, he had a number of really positive qualities. He was very intelligent, inquisitive, and creative, and he was really good with tasks that required spatial design. He was also quite strong-willed, which I tend to really like in kids, but, obviously, that also worked against him (and us), as we shall see.

Lucas's parents had tried valiantly to secure mental health services for him over the years. He was placed into two virtual individualized outpatient programs (IOP), and one brief residential program. Curiously, he had been seeing the same individual therapist virtually for the previous three years, but he attended those sessions only about half the time. Lucas would often be very nonchalant about missing a session, stating that he'd forgotten or overslept. His parents were still responsible for paying for the missed sessions, which was understandably a source of great irritation for them.

In hindsight, we can see why each of these mental health services was doomed to failure. If exposure therapy is what Lucas needed, how in the world could a virtual IOP program do him a bit of good? The residential program might have had some value, as it got him out of the house and put him in a situation in which he really had no choice but to interact with others. Unfortunately, though, he told his parents that he was miserable there and so they took him out. However, I am most perplexed by his individual therapist. I have no idea what they talked about in therapy for three years, but it clearly wasn't helping, as it was during this same time period that Lucas's functioning progressively worsened. His therapist probably correctly talked to him about doing some exposure exercises, but I'm sure he refused to do any of them.

The problem was not what was happening on the inside of Lucas; the problem was what was happening on the outside. The treatment he really needed, exposure work, was not taking place because, under his current circumstances, no one could get him to do it.

My colleagues and I knew this was going to be a challenging case because right off the bat there were several situational influences that were going to make our work much harder.

The first was how long Lucas had been housebound. We could make a reasonable guess that he would likely do better with in-person sessions, and just getting him out of the house for that reason alone would be a form of exposure therapy. He was mostly agreeable to treatment, but I find many anxious-avoidant kids are, at least at first. Their previous therapists generally have not placed many demands on them, so it was easy for the kid to show up for a session but then not do any actual work. It was also easy for them to leave a session early, either because the therapist had said something mildly challenging and had held them somewhat accountable ("I've noticed you've talked a lot about wanting to feel better, but you're not doing any of things that will make that happen"). They might also just simply leave the session on a whim, especially if the session was virtual. We tried our best to get Lucas to agree to come to our office (the family's home was too far away for us to travel there), but that was a non-starter for him, so we were stuck with virtual sessions for the duration of his care.

Lucas did, in fact, start off by attending his sessions. He did somewhat better with his weekly individual therapy and skills training sessions, but, even then, he was often late to session and his parents needed to coax him quite a bit to log on. Family therapy was a lot harder for Lucas, however, as it often is for many of the kids we treat. I think Lucas was completely unaccustomed to having meaningful, extended conversations with his parents about harder topics, because when the family tried to do so at home, he would employ various strategies to bring the conversation to a close (arguing, getting mad, walking away, shutting down, and so on). This is a lot harder for kids to do with a therapist present who will be setting some reasonable limits on their behavior in session. For example, we will disrupt argumentativeness: "Wait, wait, hold on ..." and ask family members to speak gently to each other and listen without interrupting. So, when the behaviors Lucas was accustomed to employing to avoid conversations with his parents (and being held accountable for his behavior to some degree), he was left with the only two strategies at his disposal: Leave the session early or simply not come at all. Lucas most often chose the latter.

Attending sessions, therefore, was a problem that we needed to deal with almost right away. Interestingly, we have learned that kids do not need to buy into treatment fully for treatment to still be highly effective. It's a bit counterintuitive but it's true. We prefer that kids buy in, obviously, and things progress more quickly when this is the case, but we can still bring about significant improvement. In IFFT, when a kid is reluctant to participate, we begin with gentle, friendly persuasion, which includes a healthy dose of humor and warmth. We are super easy with kids and hope they come around, as most of them eventually do. We are quite patient as well, and in Lucas's case, this is all we did for the first several months. Sometimes he would attend and sometimes he wouldn't, but we were hoping with this approach alone over time, we'd warm him up enough so that he'd participate at least somewhat willingly.

However, that's not what happened. His attendance actually got worse over time, so we knew we'd need to change course, and soon.

Since we hypothesized that time on his device was a chief contributor to his anxious avoidance, this seemed like as good a time as any to begin disrupting its influence on him. We also needed somehow to get Lucas to attend his sessions, so we wanted an incentive powerful enough to overcome his avoidance. It is important to note that it would be inaccurate to attribute all of Lucas's avoidance of therapy to anxiety alone, as this was clearly not the case. Lucas could often be quite stubborn, and he would simply refuse to do anything he just didn't want to do. To some degree, this was developmentally normal as Lucas was approaching 18. No older adolescent likes to be told what to do by their parents, so some of his behavior was quite understandable. As kids move into their later adolescent years, there is an increasingly strong need for independence and autonomy. Yet, in many cases, this need clashes with the fact that many kids do not have the wisdom or maturity to navigate this part of their lives in healthy ways. They want to be able to make their own decisions, but often those decisions are not very good ones. Therefore, when parents of older teens step in and set limits out of necessity, fireworks often ensue. I should note as well that, in my experience, most avoidant kids are also at least somewhat oppositional so they often require limit setting from their parents (making their expectations of the child clear and using reasonable consequences if these expectations are not met).

Lucas's strong-willed nature, coupled with his age and his strong avoidance, were key ingredients in what was going so terribly wrong in this family. So, how do you get an avoidant, sometimes stubborn, kid to do something they don't want to do, even when it's in their best interests to do it? You give them a reason, that's how. Time to start leveraging his devices.

That, however, leads us to the next problem with this family that needs our attention.

I spoke in the previous chapter about how loving, well-intentioned parents can contribute to their child's anxiety, and this was especially true with this family. Despite all of the great qualities Lucas's parents had, limit setting was not one of them. I've noticed that for many parents, setting limits is just not their natural strength. Good parenting requires many different strengths, such as being affectionate, attentive, warm, kind, flexible, and so on. Lucas's parents had all these skills in abundance. However, kids also need limits set for them, so they have a clear understanding of their parent's authority and understand what the world expects of them relative to their behavior.

There was a younger sibling in the house too, whose behavior could be very extreme, often bullying the parents and speaking to them in highly disrespectful ways. In a sense, both kids were a mismatch to their parents. If both kids were less strong-willed, things would have been much better, or, conversely, if the parents were stronger limit setters, again things in this family would have been much better.

In truth, both kids had been taught by their parents to be explosive. By taught, I mean that their behavior was inadvertently reinforced many times over the years, so both kids learned (unconsciously) that getting angry worked. No one enjoys interacting with an angry, explosive teenager, so it's easy to fall into the habit of acquiescing to their demands just to calm them down. However, this is the worst thing a parent could possibly do in this situation, as there is no better recipe for creating a young tyrant (or an adult tyrant for that matter). Standing one's ground and enforcing reasonable expectations can be difficult, understandably, but the message that needs to be sent to kids is that they may not like what they're being asked to do, but they still need to do it anyway. Again, I'm only talking about reasonable things, like helping out around the house, being kind, doing their homework, and so on. Obviously, it's not okay for parents to be tyrants either. In addition, for kids who get explosive, the message that needs to be communicated is that they can be as mad as they like, being mad is a normal part of life, but refusing to do reasonable things or screaming at their parents is not okay, even if they have a mental health condition.

Therefore, to get Lucas to his sessions, we were going to need to leverage his laptop. By leverage, I mean use it to incentivize him to attend his sessions by giving him access to it only when he attends. We were reasonably confident this would be effective, but how did we get parents who weren't great limit setters to set what was sure to be a difficult limit? And, even if we could pull this off with the parents, how would we safely navigate the explosion that we predicted would occur based on what we knew about Lucas?

To add another layer of complexity, Lucas did not begin by exploding; he began by persuading. He's a very smart and quite verbal kid. And fast too, my goodness. His parents sent me an audio recording of an argument that took place over asking him to move something from the living room to his bedroom. I must say, I was very impressed by Lucas's skills. He must have thrown a dozen arguments at his parents, one right after the other. They were good ones too, such as "Doesn't this house belong to all of us?" and "Almost everything in the living room belongs to you, so why can't I have just a few things here too?" Lucas's parents, being the kind people they were, would respond to each argument one by one, but I could hear them become flustered. They could barely respond to one argument before Lucas came up with another, so the entire exchange ended up going nowhere.

I encourage parents never to argue with their kids because most of the time it ends up in a tug-of-war, usually with both sides becoming angry. I tell parents that, by definition, it's only an argument when two people are speaking. If one side goes quiet, then what remains is a kid up on a soapbox just giving a speech. Another good line that I learned from the late therapist James Lehman is, "You don't have to attend every argument you're invited to." [Note: *The best response when a kid argues with you about not wanting to do something is to say, "Look, I know you don't want to do it, but I'm not going to argue with you about it. Thanks for taking care of that," and then turn around and walk away. If they still don't do what was asked, you can say what I refer to as an "if/then statement," something like: "If you expect to be on your phone later today (or your tablet, or see your friends this weekend, etc.) then I suggest you get it done, but I'll let you decide on that."* No raised voices, no angry tone—*just say it in a confident and matter-of-fact way and let the contingency (the potential loss of the phone or whatever) do the persuading for you.]*

Before we could get Lucas to his sessions, we needed to lay the groundwork with his parents knowing that they were the only ones in the system who had enough power to pull this off. We began with the limit-setting side of things. First, I spent a lot of time talking with them about why this was important, and how the absence of limit setting, and acquiescing to Lucas when he didn't want to do things was playing a very big part in his current issues. They understood this on an intellectual level, but they very much struggled in the execution. The parents needed quite a lot of encouragement and support, and I gave them time and space to decide when they were ready to begin trying something new. In this case, it was very helpful that they had a team of therapists supporting them, and knowing we were available after hours for coaching and support helped build their confidence as well.

Okay, so step one completed—Lucas's parents were on board with setting the limits around attending therapy sessions, and agreed to restrict Lucas's access to devices should he choose not to attend. *[Note: The easiest way to restrict access to a laptop is to configure one's Internet router to identify that particular device and disable its access remotely so you don't have to physically take the device away. Remotely restricting access to a phone is a little more complicated but can still easily be done. I never recommend that parents physically take a device from a child because that can go wrong in countless ways.]*

Step two in the process was teaching Lucas's parents how to stop arguing with him. It was a certainty that when he was told he'd lose access to his laptop, he would make every attempt possible to talk them out of it. It was, after all, what he was accustomed to doing so it was sure to happen. As I mentioned, Lucas was a fabulous arguer, so his parents needed a lot of practice on how not to argue in return. I suspected too, as many avoidant kids do, he would go right to the heartstrings on this one: "Why are you doing this to me? I'll do therapy when I'm ready, I told you. Therapy makes me even more anxious, is that what you want? How is it good for me not to talk to my friends? It's good for my depression." Again, the simplest and most effective response is: "I know you don't agree but we're doing this anyway."

As I mentioned in the previous chapter, kids will never agree with this plan so let go of trying to persuade them. His parents had already spoken to him endlessly about the value of therapy, but remember he's scared (hence the avoidance), with a healthy dose of stubbornness mixed in too.

Combine all that with the principle of least effort and you have what you have. Lucas is operating under numerous incentives not to see the value of therapy, so let go of trying to convince him. When parents set a limit, and to reduce the probability of an extended argument, it is best to keep the conversation to about two minutes or less. Argumentative kids will happily take whatever amount of time is afforded them to argue. Give them an hour, and they'll take an hour. Parents often fall into the trap of arguing for hours on end with their kids when, in most cases, an expectation or limit can be set in just minutes.

Learning how to set limits differently and side-step arguments, especially if these are not part of a parent's skill set, takes time and practice. I spend quite a lot of time in my parent sessions roleplaying and practicing these skills until I feel like the parents have them down. I'll start by playing the part of the parent to demonstrate what to say and how to say it and ask them to play the part of their kid. I ask them to say everything their child or teen might say to them in that situation, and I give them my full permission to come at me hard. I teach them not just the words to say, but the tone, body language, and facial expressions to accompany the words (relaxed, matter-of-fact, and confident). We do that a few times and then we switch. I play the part of the kid and ask them to try to set the limit with me, and I throw everything I can at the parent. I do this over and over, with both parents, until I feel they've got it down.

In the case of Lucas, that conversation about therapy flowed like this:

Parents (P):   So, we've talked with you quite a few times about the importance of therapy, but you're still not going, yes?

Lucas (L):   Therapy doesn't work, I told you that.
[This is what I call a "red herring," a distraction of sorts. Kids often throw out red herrings that take a variety of forms, all of which are intended to distract from the real topic at hand. He could just as easily have said, "Therapy makes me feel worse," or "I'll go to therapy, but I want a different therapist." To be fair to Lucas, his statement of therapy not working is completely true, or at least so far. I encourage parents never to respond directly to a red herring because that just provides an incentive for more red herrings, making it impossible to stick to the topic at hand.]

P: We're not here to talk about those things today. *[Notice they don't respond at all to "therapy doesn't work and they just keep going."]* We also realize that trying to persuade you to go to your sessions hasn't worked so we're not doing that today. But, because we love you, we also can't just sit by and do nothing. You have a session this afternoon and

	we expect you to go to it. And all of your other sessions after that too, please.
L:	I told you I won't do therapy until I feel ready.
P:	Well, go or don't go, that's up to you. If you don't though, we're disabling your Internet access for the remainder of that day and the day after.
L:	You can't do that.
P:	We can. Starting today.
L:	It's my laptop! That's not fair. If you really loved me, you wouldn't make me do something that makes me worse.
P:	Well, nevertheless, we are. And now this conversation is over.

I cannot see how that even took two minutes, barely one probably. And now, Lucas is going to react in a big way because his parents have changed the rules of the game. They are behaving in a way that he's unaccustomed to, and when this happens, kids will double down on whatever behavior they have learned over the years to get what they want. It's good to prepare parents for this so they can anticipate it, otherwise, they might incorrectly conclude what they did has made things worse. When parents change course and start to set limits in a different way, it usually takes several weeks for a child or teen's behavior to start to improve, so it's also good to let parents know this too.

Lucas is not a bad kid; he's a scared kid. He almost certainly has no awareness or understanding as to why he behaves the way he does; he's just playing out his part in the family dance.

We knew that we also needed to attend to safety in the home if Lucas's parents were going to start leveraging his device. This was the third problem that needed to be solved by the team, as it was understandably a concern for the parents, as well as one of their chief incentives for not setting better limits over the years. We knew from Lucas's history that when he escalated and became enraged, he had never become physically aggressive toward anyone. He did some property damage, but it tended to be somewhat on the milder side (throwing a glass to the floor, for example). A yelling kid who sometimes breaks things, while not ideal, can be ignored. *[Side note: We advise parents to never stay engaged (talk with) a kid who is angry and disrespectful. Doing so is counterproductive as it typically just keeps them in an agitated state even longer. They need time to cool off and re-regulate, and they are far more likely to do so when parents stop talking to them. I do not feel it is a parent's responsibility to help a kid cool off; it's the kid's job to do that. It gives the child or teen the opportunity to learn how to regulate their emotions themselves rather than relying on others in their environment to do that for them. It's best for a parent to just say, "I can't talk with you when you're yelling and saying unkind things to me. Happy to talk once you've calmed down." It is far more effective for parents only to pay attention to kids once they've calmed down and are more respectful. Over time, the child learns that the only way to get and hold their parents' attention is when they are emotionally regulated and being reasonable.]*

Lucas's history was not to become physically aggressive, but as we all know, history doesn't always accurately predict future behavior. However, it's a good starting place, and that's all we had. We knew the upsets would come, so we planned accordingly. I spent a lot of time coaching the parents on what to do and say in that moment, and how to disengage and walk away from him. I also advised the parents that if Lucas did become physically aggressive, they should leave the house or call law enforcement. I do not advise involving law enforcement in every case, and definitely not with younger children, but given Lucas's age, this seemed appropriate. I also reminded the parents that they could reach out to the team at any time if Lucas's behavior escalated and they were unsure as to how to respond.

Again, no parent should attempt to use this type of strategy on their own without professional help.

Leveraging Lucas's laptop worked. He got mad the first time his device was turned off but I'm happy to say there was far less emotional upset than we predicted. He began to attend sessions regularly, sometimes he was slow to log in, but he still did it. In fact, we generally find this works quite well in just about every family. Leveraging phones and devices is an effective strategy, not just to get a child or teen to attend sessions, but also to motivate them to engage in their sessions in a reasonable way. Some kids, when they've been told they'll lose their devices for a while if they don't go to therapy, will go to the session, but all they'll do is show up—not a lot else. They will give one-word answers to questions, look and sound annoyed, and so on. When this happens, we ask their parents to tell them that therapy is more than just walking in the door, it's also participating to a reasonable degree, and this works quite well.

Someone reading this might reasonably ask what good is "forcing" a reluctant kid to do therapy? It does a world of good, actually. Every therapist prefers a willing client, but the reality of working with challenging kids is that they often just aren't all that willing. I think it's a combination of not really knowing what therapy entails, thinking that if they go to therapy there really must be something wrong with them, or that their parents are to blame so why is it fair that they get stuck with therapy? When viewed from this perspective, a child or adolescent's reluctance makes a lot of sense, I think. The problem is, even the best treatments won't help a kid if they avoid treatment altogether. Here is what is important to know about this: Almost all kids eventually warm up to the therapy even when at first they really don't want to be there. They slowly start to engage, get to know and like their therapist, and then big changes happen. And, as I mentioned before, even for the rare kid who never fully engages, great progress can still be made because we are also working on many other important aspects of the family system, as well as mitigating negative social influences and other situational variables.

Was it Lucas's preference that, as he suggested, we wait until he "felt better" to start treatment and not put pressure on him to engage in therapy? Absolutely. I'm reasonably confident, however, that we'd still be waiting to this day while his functioning and mood deteriorated more and more.

We leveraged Lucas's device not just to get him to attend his sessions, but we also used that strategy to incentivize him to do just about everything else he was disinclined to do. By month four of treatment, he had resumed bathing, brushing his teeth most days, and doing chores around the house. Lucas would still intermittently refuse, but this was not due to anxiety. It was clearly more about an older teenager just not wanting to be told what to do. Lucas and his parents were able to fall into an easy rhythm on this without a lot of fireworks and upset. For example, if he refused to do a chore or take a shower, his parents would just turn off his Wi-Fi access until he did. He might hold out for a day or two, but rarely longer. On occasion, Lucas would find a way to get around the Wi-Fi restrictions through some clever technological means, but it was obvious to his parents when he did so, and they would regain control of his access without a lot of fanfare.

Also in month four of treatment, despite the fact he was not currently attending school (he hadn't for years), Lucas's school sent a nice basket to the house congratulating him on successfully graduating from high school. This was about as tone-deaf as it gets and very upsetting to his parents, understandably. (I'm assuming his school did this as a matter of course for seniors, but it might be a good idea to make sure the kid actually graduated before sending out a basket.)

Lucas's mood gradually started to improve as he started to do more. Prior to the start of treatment, we asked him why he thought his life had stalled out and he said, "I'm depressed so I'm not motivated to do anything." I think there is truth in that. Since he could not come up with the motivation himself to overcome his avoidance, his parents needed to provide that motivation externally, which was really all he needed. Lucas also attributed his low mood to sleep apnea, but I do not think his sleeping problems were about that (he had a device to help with apnea, but he never used it). The sleep issues resolved quickly when his parents started to disable his Internet access at 9:00 p.m. each night, at which time his sleep/awake cycle normalized.

Lucas also started to come out of his room and spend quite a bit more time with his family. This change happened naturally without any sort of intervention on our part. This can probably be attributed to the reduction in tension between Lucas and his parents as there was a lot less to argue about. As we do with every family, we also taught the parents how to look for examples of positive behavior and comment on them (reinforce them) with a statement such as "I love how quickly you got your chores done today. It's impressive what a hard worker you are."

Lucas's individual and family sessions were going smoothly by month five, for the most part anyway. He was generally willing to attend, and when in session he was reasonably open and communicative. This allowed his therapists to spend quite a lot of time talking about the role avoidance plays in the development and maintenance of anxiety, and how stepping into anxiety-provoking situations will, over time, reduce his anxiety. They also taught Lucas a variety of skills and anxiety-management strategies, but in truth, these were less valuable to his treatment than just creating an environment that made it much harder for him to engage in avoidant behavior. On occasion, Lucas would still refuse to do a session, but this generally occurred when he was mad at his parents for something. When this occurred, they would just quietly turn off his Wi-Fi access until he attended his next scheduled session.

At month five, Lucas's parents and the treatment team felt it was time to tackle going back to school. By this point, Lucas was on a roll, and this required surprisingly little effort on the part of his parents or the team. Lucas's parents just sat down with him one day and floated the idea of going back to school. Much to everyone's surprise and delight, he was agreeable. They settled on a hybrid program—some online independent study, but also two days per week on campus. We were expecting some trouble on this as Lucas had been out of school for years, but thankfully trouble never came, and the return to high school went without a hitch. Lucas made the comment, "I feel better about myself now that I'm finishing classes." In fact, he finished so many classes that he was able to graduate from high school by the end of that calendar year.

By month nine, the family was able to take a week-long family vacation.

During month ten, while things were still generally going well, there was some backsliding. Lucas missed a day or two of school, and, on occasion, he wouldn't get up on time for class. These types of issues were usually brief, however, and most of the time he would get back on track all on his own.

After high school, Lucas had so much positive momentum that he took on two new challenges: He enrolled in college classes (some online, some in person, and he was able to get a part-time job at a local retail chain stocking shelves. Lucas would still mention his anxiety, but generally in passing only, and he never missed a day of work.

Clinical Outcomes

As I mentioned in Chapter 8, it is very important to us that we measure whether a patient and their family improves over the course of treatment, and if so, to what degree. I have already described the two measures that we use, the Youth Outcomes Questionnaire (Y-OQ2.01), which is a standardized measure of behavior change, and the Child & Adolescent Family Functioning Inventory (CAFFI), which measures improvement in family functioning (ability to solve problems, managing conflict, closeness and connection, and so on). I will refer the reader back to Chapter 8 for a more detailed discussion of both measures, but I'll summarize their key elements here. [*Note: We did not collect data on Lucas's scores mid-way through treatment as we did with Maricela (it was just an oversight). So, for our purposes here, we can only compare his scores at the start of treatment with his scores at its conclusion.*]

A quick reminder on the Y-OQ The measure produces a total score, with higher scores indicating a greater degree of clinical and behavioral impairment. A total score of 47 or greater is considered the clinical cutoff (more than that and the child or adolescent has significant problems), and the goal of treatment is to reduce the total score as close to the normal range as possible (the community, or nonclinical sample, of 23.3 or less). The average total score of children and teens in inpatient settings (psychiatric hospitals) is 110, and for kids in residential treatment programs, it is 115.

Lucas's Y-OQ scores over the course of treatment can be seen in Figure 11.1.

Not quite as high as Maricela's intake Y-OQ score in the previous case example, but Lucas's total score at the start of treatment (114) was still quite high. It is very close to the same mean Y-OQ total score for kids in residential treatment (recall he had been in residential treatment before we started work with this family) and above the average score of teens inpatient (in psychiatric hospitals; 110). At the conclusion of treatment, Lucas's Y-OQ total score had dropped down significantly to a score of 53. This was still above the clinical cutoff of 47, but it is very close so in the end we were content with that and so was his family.

A reminder on the CAFFI: It is completed by the parents, and scores reflect their perceptions of how well their family functions within five treatment domains. Higher scores on the CAFFI indicate poorer family functioning. A family's scores on the CAFFI are compared with a normative (nonclinical) sample, with the goal of treatment to lower the family's scores to as close to the normal range as possible. Lucas's five CAFFI scores over the course of treatment (intake and discharge) are compared with a nonclinical sample in Figure 11.2.

Lucas's Y-OQ Scores

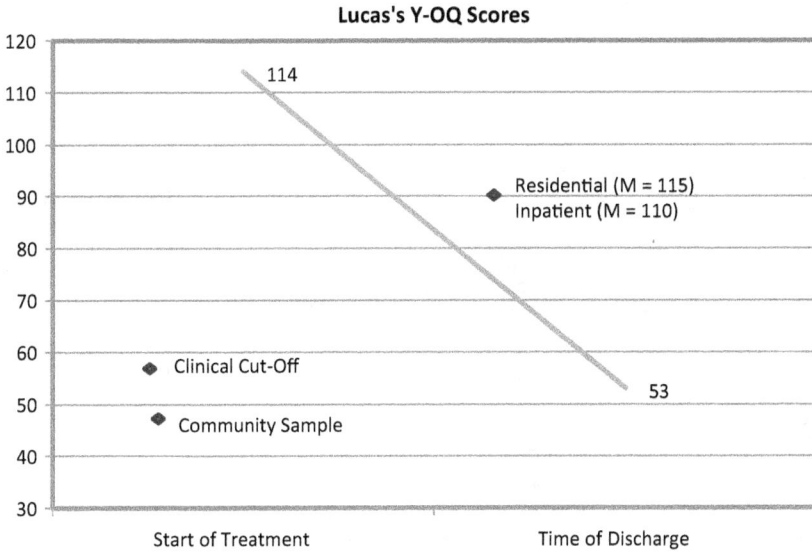

Figure 11.1 Lucas's scores on the Y-OQ at intake and at the time of discharge.

Lucas's CAFFI Subscale Scores

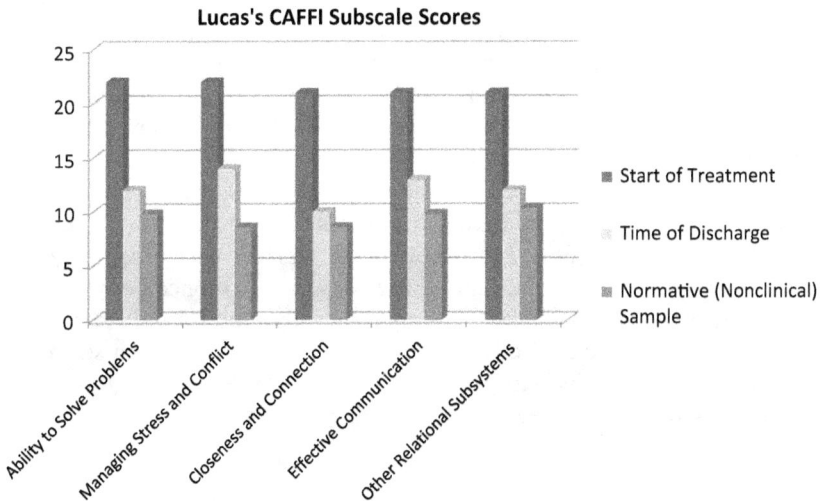

Figure 11.2 Lucas's scores on the five CAFFI subscales at intake and at the time of discharge in comparison to a normative (nonclinical) sample.

Lucas's CAFFI Total Scores

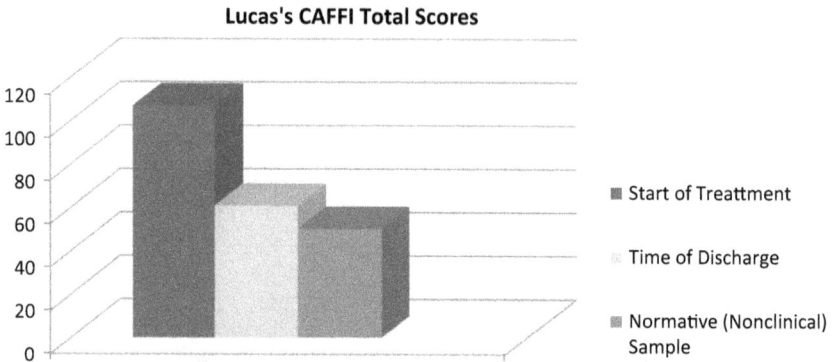

Figure 11.3. Lucas's total scores on the CAFFI at intake and at the time of discharge in comparison to a normative (nonclinical) sample.

In addition, his intake and discharge total scores over the course of treatment in comparison with the normative sample are shown in Figure 11.3.

As can be seen, all five of Lucas's subscale scores significantly decreased (improved) over the course of his treatment, as did his total score. While his scores improved quite a bit, they still remained somewhat higher than the nonclinical sample.

As mentioned, and as is the case with most parents of the anxious-avoidant kids my colleagues and I have treated, Lucas's parents were just a delight. They were incredibly warm and compassionate people who wanted the very best for their son, and there was never any doubt about that. Despite everyone's good intentions, the entire family had become stuck in a situation no one wanted, but which no one knew how to change.

By the end of treatment, Lucas was far more engaged in life, and consequently, as we would predict, his mood was also greatly improved. As I have described throughout this book, we started with changing his behavior first and not his mood, because we knew that once he started to move forward again in life, improvements in his mood would naturally follow. That is, in fact, exactly what happened, as it does with so many children and adolescents with mental health challenges.

Once kids do better, they feel better. It's as simple as that.

Part IV

Directions for the Future

12 An 18-Item, Research-Informed Strategy for Reversing the Childhood Mental Health Crisis

In this final chapter, I am going to bring together the most important elements of the book and make some very specific recommendations to parents, therapists, school counselors, and health insurance companies for improving the lives and treatment of children and adolescents with mental health conditions. Given that the rates of depression, anxiety, and suicide/self-harm continue to increase, I think it is safe to say that what we are doing is not working particularly well. I firmly believe we can do better, and must, but to do so is going to require a shift in how all of us—parents and providers alike—respond to the mental health crisis among our children.

The late clinical psychologist Paul Meehl, famously critical of the profession of psychotherapy, wrote "If you want to shake people up, you have to raise a little hell" (Meehl, 1973). It is not my intention to raise hell, necessarily, or to be unduly critical, but it absolutely is my intention to disrupt the current mental health system as it pertains to children and teens. I strongly believe that parents and their children are not getting what they need or deserve and that they have often been led astray by the very professionals who have been entrusted to provide care.

Please note, however, that with just a few exceptions, every therapist, psychiatrist, and school counselor that I have met is very well-intentioned. This is not about a lack of compassion or clinical skill; that is not the issue. Therapists, by and large, are good at what we do, but we also tend to be a bit myopic—we see things through the lens of what we have been taught or a particular treatment we currently favor, but we are not always as well-dialed into other ways of looking at things, often to the detriment of children and families. There are countless examples of this. Therapists trained in DBT see the world through that lens and intervene accordingly, as is the case with a CBT therapist. Psychiatrists tend to see and treat mental illness from a biological perspective and prescribe medications intended to improve how a patient's brain functions. Some therapists see a patient's struggles through a trauma lens and direct their treatment interventions in ways they believe will help patients process traumatic experiences.

DOI: 10.4324/9781003397366-17

What each of these treatment approaches has in common is an implicit bias: There is something wrong going on inside the child or adolescent that needs correcting. How a therapist goes about providing help generally involves directing treatment through whichever lens is most favored by the therapist, and the majority of the time, that treatment is delivered by way of individual therapy, or other therapies directed primarily or exclusively at the child. Directing treatment at the child or teen individually has merit and is essential, but in doing that alone the larger universe of external social and situational influences acting on the child are often under-appreciated, overlooked, and generally left unchanged. As I have stated earlier in the book, change the situation and you change the kid.

As I have also said throughout this book, I believe that a better way to help struggling young people is to spend more of our time, both parents and clinicians, looking at what is happening to them on the outside rather than primarily directing our attention to what is happening on the inside.

Table 12.1 lists the 18 specific strategies I am recommending for improving our community-based responses to the child and adolescent mental health crisis, and I will discuss each one in turn. Each strategy or proposed change is supported or informed by research, as well as my nearly four decades of clinical experience working with almost a thousand children and families. I hope to expand this list over time, and I welcome additions from parents, clinicians, researchers, and just about anyone else who has a good idea.

Strategies Implemented by Parents

Mitigating the Negative Effects of Phones and Other Devices

Hopefully, I have made a convincing argument that smartphones and other devices have played a key role in why so many children and teens are experiencing mental health problems. I think this hypothesis is well supported by the available evidence, such as the trend toward increased depression, anxiety, and self-harm coinciding with the year 2012 when for the first time the majority of children and teens were routinely using smartphones.

Therefore, in terms of intervening in the problem of child and adolescent mental illness, I highly recommend we begin here. The changes I am proposing are best implemented when a child gets their first phone because, in my experience, they are so eager to have it they would agree to just about anything. In general, it is much easier to start a child off with very limited and carefully monitored device usage and slowly give them more freedom earned over time than trying to wrestle those freedoms away from a kid who already has them.

However, even if your child or teen currently has unrestricted, unmonitored access to their phones and other devices, you can still step in

Table 12.1 An 18-Item, Research-Informed Strategy for Improving the Treatment of Child and Adolescent Mental Illness

Strategies and Changes Implemented by Parents
1. Reduce your child or teen's screen time (phone, tablet, etc.) to no more than about two hours per day.
2. If this is not implemented for whatever reason, consider creating 2–3 hour device-free time periods each day.
3. Electronically monitor your child's text messaging to alert you to problematic content using a third-party app such as Bark or the equivalent.
4. Phones should be completely disabled an hour or two before bed, and, ideally, not allowed in the bedroom all night.
5. Treat your child as capable, push for them to become independent, and resist the temptation to rescue and over-protect them.
6. Stay mindful of the power of language.
7. Maintain your parental authority.
8. Learn how to communicate better and solve problems in a more matter-of-fact, peaceful way.
9. Seek out a therapist who does more than just individual therapy, especially in cases of very serious mental illness.
10. Find a therapist who is knowledgeable and skilled at behavior change and can teach you how to use these techniques at home.
Strategies and Changes Implemented by the Mental Health Community
11. Family-based therapy, rather than individual therapy, should be a first-line treatment, not the second or third, especially for cases of severe mental illness.
12. Language and classifications have power for therapists too, perhaps even more so than at home. Let go of "diagnostic" labels that are not helpful.
13. Be honest and transparent about what approach you use, and its limitations.
14. For school counselors: Capitalize on parents far more often, and, despite good intentions, be wary of interventions used on campus that are counter-productive to building resilience.
Strategies and Changes Implemented by Insurance and Healthcare Companies
15. Become knowledgeable about, and capitalize on, the almost 40 years of research documenting the efficacy of family therapy.
16. Assign a care advocate to families to keep patients from being shuffled from one unhelpful treatment to another.
17. Consider incentivizing family therapists so that there are more of us.
18. Parents are scared, so treat them like human beings.

and begin to regulate them. Kids will protest and argue about it, of course, but it is entirely doable, and I know this because I work with parents who pull it off every day. If your child is explosive or engages in unsafe behavior, you are going to need professional help with this, but I promise you it can be done.

Additionally, I also highly recommend that you do not wait for the government to pass legislation to compel the tech industry to make your child's devices safer. Given how slowly this is moving, I suspect your children will be grandparents by the time this finally happens in any meaningful way. You can do this yourself once you decide it is time to do so.

1. Reduce your child or teen's screen time (phone, tablet, etc.) to no more than a couple of hours per day. Problems this intervention addresses: Dose-related effect; social and emotional contagion; echo chambers; kids isolating in their bedrooms; and the crowding-out effect.

As you will recall from Chapter 1, for every additional hour a child or teen spends on a phone, there is a 13% increased risk of depression. Moods are socially contagious, meaning if kids are interacting with other depressed and anxious kids, they are far more likely to become depressed and anxious themselves. Behaviors are socially contagious as well. Most children and teens know at least one classmate who hurts themselves, and just the mere fact of routinely interacting with others and talking about self-harm, anxiety, school avoidance, and so on is a risk factor for engaging in that same behavior. "Echo chambers" strengthen this further by reinforcing dysfunctional behaviors within closed groups. Crowding out refers to how excessive time on devices makes it harder for kids to engage in other wellness-enhancing behaviors, such as interacting with family, engaging in sports, going outside, doing homework, and so on. A couple of hours a day on a device is plenty and probably within the margin of safety, especially for younger kids (although your child will loudly disagree with me on this but that's okay).

Through various third-party apps, phones and tablets can be well controlled remotely by parents and configured in ways that make it very difficult for kids to disable the restrictions. I recommend limiting screen time by setting timers that automatically disable the device at specified times (parents often forget to manually disable devices at the agreed-upon time and kids, of course, never remind them to turn them off). In IFFT, we always recommend that parents obtain the ability to disable their child's phone remotely rather than asking for the phone itself. This reduces the probability of an argument and perhaps even a scuffle. (I do not recommend that you try to wrestle a phone away from an angry kid as that can go south quickly).

2. If this is not implemented for whatever reason, consider creating 2–3 hour device-free time periods each day. Problems this intervention addresses: As above.

Device-free time periods are my second choice over vastly reducing screen time, but this approach also works quite well. Device-free time periods are for the entire family and not just the kid. It is a set period of an hour or two on weeknights and three or four hours on the weekend in which no one in the family uses a device. Kids will again protest this, but usually within a couple of weeks the protests fade away and they settle into the routine of it. Magically, once kids have nothing to do in their bedrooms and parents are no longer in competition with a device, kids begin to wander out in search of something to do, which often involves interacting with family members. Increased time with family (assuming that time is peaceful) is, in my opinion, one of the essential ingredients in helping kids get well again. I have used the term *family is medicine* and I really do see it that way. When kids reconnect and build strong relationships with their parents, that becomes a powerful antidote to depression and anxiety.

Electronically monitor your child's text messaging to alert you to problematic content, using a third-party app such as Bark or the equivalent. Problems this intervention addresses: Behavioral and emotional contagion; not knowing whether your child or teen is engaging in high-risk conversations and/or behavior.

I believe monitoring your child or teen's online activity and messaging is essential, especially if they engage in self-harming or other high-risk behaviors. Teens often reveal plans of suicide to their peers well before anyone else. Monitoring their exchanges also allows parents the ability to disrupt negative peer influences and echo chambers, as well as protect children and teens from interacting with adult predators. Bark is useful in that it still affords kids some privacy. It alerts parents to content only by identifying key words that are problematic, such as "suicide," "cutting," "getting high," and so on.

Phones should be completely disabled an hour or two before bed, and, ideally, not allowed in the bedroom all night. Problems this intervention addresses: Inadequate sleep; late-night conversations with peers that are worrisome, unhelpful, or problematic.

It cannot be overstated the role that sleep deprivation plays in childhood mental health problems. Kids just generally do not get enough sleep, usually because they are up late at night communicating with peers. Devices are made to be addictive, and, consequently, it is the rare child or adolescent who can put their phone down early enough at night to get a good night's sleep. They simply need their parents' help with this, and while they will not like turning in their phones at night at first, it will do them the world of good. Restricting phones at night also keeps kids from having conversations into the early morning hours about topics that are not good for them. Any online conversation at 2:00 a.m. is unlikely a helpful one. I find it is best for phones and tablets to be out of the bedroom completely so the temptation to send or respond to a text is reduced further (not to mention reducing the amount of time a kid has available to circumvent the restrictions).

Foster Resiliency and Independence

Treat your child as capable, push for them to become independent, and resist the temptation to rescue and over-protect them. Problems this intervention addresses: Counteracts the principle of least effort; increases resilience; promotes healthy independence; builds self-esteem; and assumes kids are capable human beings rather than sending them the message that they are "damaged goods" ("falling into the pool").

The current generation of children and teens (Gen Z and Gen Alpha) have never been kept safer due to a cultural shift that emphasizes protection and adult oversight (so-called "helicopter" parenting). However, this shift may have brought with it a degree of over-protection that is depriving kids of opportunities to build the age-appropriate independence that was expected of previous generations. Kids have become more dependent than ever on their parents, and research indicates there may be an association between this dependence and the rapid increase in depression, anxiety, and suicide. This trend can be counteracted in part by holding children and teens accountable for all of the normal, age-typical responsibilities of life, such as doing chores around the house, getting their driver's license, and getting a part-time job. Set high expectations for your child's capabilities rather than setting low ones.

It is very common for kids with mental health conditions to gradually do less and less by convincing their parents they are no longer capable of meeting age-typical responsibilities. Parents who are highly susceptible to this ask less and less of them ("falling into the pool," i.e., agreeing that their "condition" prevents them from doing things that are hard). I have learned from experience that when parents set the bar of expectations low for their kids, kids might hit that low bar but often go no higher. Children and teens develop self-esteem and confidence by doing hard things and mastering them, not by avoiding them, and certainly not by being excused from normal responsibilities. By giving your kids opportunities to try, including opportunities in which they might fail, you are fostering resilience and creating strong, capable adults, not fragile, dependent ones. We grow and evolve in hard spaces, not the easy ones.

Stay mindful of the power of language. Problems this intervention addresses: The classification effect; unconscious expectancy; and "falling into the pool."

Language has a great deal of power to influence our perception of situations and events. The words that we use to frame an experience go a long way in determining what that experience will actually be like. Increasingly, the language that was previously used only by mental health professionals has spread to the general public and to children (e.g., "traumatic"), but in ways that are not always helpful. When an authority figure (like a therapist) tells us we have a "disorder," that creates an unconscious expectancy. We then, in turn, often behave or experience things in ways that are consistent with that classification (more on the classification effect in just a bit).

It is important for parents to be cautious in their word choice so that their child's experience is not inadvertently or unnecessarily amplified. Using words like "depressed" "anxious," or "traumatic" can often be replaced by words that in many cases actually better describe the experience, such as "feeling down," "nervous," or "upsetting." A slight variation in word choice can reduce the intensity of how an event is experienced, as well as normalize everyday feelings without pathologizing them. I feel it is important to talk to your kids like parents, not like therapists. I find once parents shift their language as I have described here, kids will often start using the more normalized language as well, probably without a conscious awareness that they have started doing so.

Maintain your parental authority. Problems this intervention addresses: Unhelpful power imbalances; inadvertently reinforcing the very behavior you are trying to change by giving in; and mitigating the "functional" (secondary) gains to the child from their mental health symptoms.

Even if your child has a mental health condition, it is still important to hold them accountable if they are disrespectful, unkind, not following basic family rules or expectations, or not fulfilling age-appropriate responsibilities. Children want and need limits placed on their behavior. Not in an unkind, over-the-top authoritarian style, but in a kind, sometimes firm, matter-of-fact, and consistent manner. Make your expectations known and clear to your kids, and back up those expectations by imposing reasonable consequences when the expectations have not been met. Children feel safest when they know their parents are in charge. When parents back off from limit setting or stop holding their kids accountable in the ways they did prior to the development of the mental health condition, this creates a power imbalance that is confusing to them (they have the power now and know you do not). Kids know when their behavior is not acceptable and are waiting for you to do or say something about it. Having a mental health condition does not absolve kids of the basic responsibility to treat others with kindness and respect. Balanced with warmth and compassion, holding kids accountable for their behavior is an essential component to raising honorable and responsible human beings, as well as helping a child successfully move past this challenging period of their life.

Learn how to communicate better and solve problems in a more matter-of-fact, peaceful way. Problems this intervention addresses: The effects of mirroring and matching; reducing tugs-of-war; and allowing you to model and maintain the high moral ground.

If you are a parent and you are reading this book, you likely have a more difficult-to-parent child than average who often behaves in ways that are quite challenging and often upsetting. I firmly believe that we never have to raise our voices to kids or speak to them harshly in order for them to do what is asked. Raising your voice in anger or frustration is rarely helpful and teaches your child to do the same thing in return (through the principle of mirroring and matching). By modeling patience and regulating our own emotions, we show kids how to communicate and solve problems in the manner in which we would like them to do so. You cannot ask your child or teen to stay well-regulated and respectful if you are not behaving that way yourself. Yelling doesn't solve problems; it just creates new ones.

Seek out a therapist who does more than just individual therapy, especially in cases of very serious mental illness. Problems this intervention addresses: Unhelpful and ineffective treatment directed solely or primarily at the child; and misdirecting attention and interventions toward the inside of what is happening with the child rather than the outside, i.e., external situational variables (isolating in their bedrooms for example) that are negatively affecting them.

I believe that family-based therapies are essential for children and adolescents with serious mental health conditions. Its benefits are well documented empirically spanning the past 40 years. However, family-based therapies are currently vastly under-utilized resources. I believe that in many cases when treatment is focused solely or primarily on the child rather than on the entire family system and other external situational influences, it is very likely going to be the wrong treatment.

A child's mental health problems are not something that exists solely within them, waiting to somehow be corrected by the right combination of therapy or medication. Far from it. Except for the few truly biologically-based disorders, such as schizophrenia or bipolar disorder, both rare in children, what we think of as "mental illness" in kids is really a combination of situational variables that are negatively impinging on their emotional well-being. Treatment involves identifying these variables and disrupting or mitigating them in ways that improve the child's mental health. Parents are the most powerful change agents in a child's life, often far more so than therapists. Change the situation and you change the kid, and parents play a vital role in that process.

Find a therapist who is knowledgeable and skilled at behavior change and can teach you how to use these techniques at home. Problems this intervention addresses: Reduces conflict and frustration; reduces behavioral challenges; and increases warmth, peace, connection, and attachment.

A large part of helping kids who struggle with a mental health condition involves changing their behavior. Kids feel better when they do better, and not the other way around. Thinking otherwise is a common mistake within my profession. No child or teen feels good about themselves when they are saying disrespectful things to their parents. Often, as therapists, we are trained to help kids feel better based on the assumption that when this happens their symptoms (largely their mood and behavior) will improve in a corresponding manner. While perhaps true in some cases, I believe this is the exception rather than the rule. It is far more effective when we teach parents how to respond to their child's behavioral challenges in ways that improve that behavior, which in turn improves their mood. Parents are hungry to learn how to do this because, in most cases, it is the child's problematic behavior that brought the family in for treatment in the first place. Not all therapists are trained in, or skilled at, behavior change, but neglecting this important area will leave most parents feeling very dissatisfied with the treatment and prolong the family's suffering.

Strategies and Changes Implemented by the Mental Health Community

I feel that in our efforts to help, the mental health community in many ways has probably made the problem of child and adolescent mental illness worse. I know many therapists would disagree with me on this, but I think it's true. We have not made it worse on purpose, of course, but many of the approaches we have adopted have made their own subtle contributions to the continued suffering of children and families.

Recommendations for Therapists

Family-based therapy, rather than individual therapy, should be a first-line treatment, not the second or third, especially for cases of severe mental illness. As I have stated throughout the book, I feel individual therapy, or individually-focused therapies alone are often insufficient to help a child or teen with a serious mental health challenge. Without adequately including the parents in treatment, a therapist is not giving adequate attention to situational variables occurring in the home or community that are likely having a profoundly negative effect on the child's well-being. If a family is having problems with communication, emotional reactivity, over- or under-utilizing consequences, and so on, the time you spend just seeing the patient alone likely will have little or no impact on these important variables. Furthermore, without involving the parents, you have only a limited ability to positively impact other situational variables that are worsening the kid's mental health, such as spending too much time on their phones, being in a relationship, or interacting with other dysfunctional peers (emotional and behavioral contagion), and not getting enough sleep. It is vital that you not overlook the people who are in the best position to help the child—their parents. If you under-capitalize on this resource, it is far more likely that the child will continue to struggle.

Additionally, to be able to help families with complex challenges, one therapist alone would need to have an extraordinarily broad skill set. The probability of finding just one therapist with the myriad skills needed to truly help distressed families is quite low. Working with a team of therapists, however, solves this problem nicely because each team member brings their own unique knowledge, skills, and abilities to the table. This enhances the strength of the treatment and mitigates the potential skills deficits of any one team member. I cannot do what my colleagues do and that goes the other way around.

Language and classifications have power for therapists too, perhaps even more so than at home. Let go of "diagnostic" labels that are not helpful. Problems this intervention addresses: The same ones it causes when parents are not mindful of language.

I think the mental health community would be wise to resist the temptation to pathologize kids and families by using unhelpful diagnostic labels. In my experience, this results in parents putting far too much emphasis on diagnosis, believing, often incorrectly, that obtaining the "right diagnosis" is going to make all the difference. In some of the more serious mental health challenges like bipolar disorder or schizophrenia, the diagnosis is helpful for medication choice and long-term treatment planning, but I rarely find it helpful for anyone else.

A "diagnosis" is really just a list of symptoms (moods and behaviors) that often cluster together, but it is the subject of longstanding debate as to whether diagnoses represent much beyond that. For example, once I had a father who asked to speak to me urgently because he stated, "I think I've figured out what's wrong with my son." When he came to see me, he handed me a list of the diagnostic criteria for oppositional defiant disorder (ODD). I had to tell him that while ODD is in the *Diagnostic and Statistical Manual of Mental Disorders* (DSM), simply picking that label to describe a kid is useless. It is just the label we use when some kids are overly stubborn and do not like to be told what to do, but it tells us nothing about why they are acting that way even less about what to do about it. In the case of this particular boy, there was nothing wrong with him per se, but there were plenty of things wrong with his situation, giving him incentive to behave in an oppositional way. His oppositional behavior, in turn, resulted in his parents responding to him in less-than-ideal ways that made him even more oppositional.

Giving a diagnosis to a person may not be as helpful as we might think; it can actually cause them harm. Earlier in the book I described the classification effect, the tendency for people, once placed into a classification, to then behave in a manner that is consistent with that classification. To tell a child or adolescent that they have "major depressive disorder" is to put them (and by extension put their parents) into a classification that is very likely going to influence their behavior in unhelpful ways. Earlier in the book, I used the example of seasonal affective disorder (SAD), which could very well be a myth given the evidence that low mood appears unrelated to the time of year. In naming this "disorder" and proclaiming someone has it, we create an expectancy within a person that their mood will decline as the winter months approach. Rather than telling a child or teen that they have a medical disorder (depression), I think it is far more appropriate to say, "I see that your mood is low sometimes, let's figure out what we can do that might help with that." (I am not saying that major depressive disorder doesn't exist, just that it is far less common among kids than one might think.)

In her excellent book, *Sleeping Beauties*, Suzanne O'Sullivan discusses the temptation to over-medicalize human suffering:

> In Western society, when things are going badly for a person, medical explanations are often sought because they are found to be more palatable than psychosocial explanations. Western medicine has, in a sense, learned to comply with the needs of the people. Thus, the lines between behavior and illness, normal and abnormal—even the demarcation between disease and health—have become so blurred that it is possible to give an illness category to almost every person. Once that is done, a person becomes a patient. (O'Sullivan, 2021, p. 291)

I tell parents it is not that I am unconcerned with diagnosis, it's that I'd much rather spend my time and theirs getting to work actually solving their family's problems.

Be honest and transparent about what approach you use, and its limitations. Problems this intervention addresses: Misleading parents into thinking they are getting a specific treatment when they might not be; creating false hopes; unnecessarily delaying the onset of a more effective treatment; and a possible "voltage drop."

A significant problem in the mental health community is a lack of transparency in our work that often misleads our patients and creates false hopes. We offer various different lettered therapies (e.g., CBT, DBT, ACT, EMDR, and so on), but families really have little or no idea what these actually are. As a profession, I believe we are not particularly good at educating parents on the various strengths and limitations of these treatments such that they can make a truly informed decision before choosing one for their child.

The term "evidenced-based treatment" has become popular in the field of clinical psychology. For many decades, my profession has paid scant attention to whether the various forms of therapy that have been developed are actually effective. I know this probably sounds strange to some readers, parents especially, but it's true. Part of the problem was that therapy outcomes could not be measured easily until more recently when various standardized psychological tests were developed (for example, tests to measure the severity of depression, anxiety, and so on). Rightfully so, the professions of clinical psychology and psychiatry were under fire for taking people's money without really knowing whether anyone was really getting better, and, if so, to what degree. The professions began to change in response to this perfectly reasonable criticism, and so, currently, it is common practice for the developers of treatment models to study their outcomes in a scientific way and publish these results in peer-reviewed, academic journals. The term "evidence-based," therefore, means that a reasonable body of research exists in which, under controlled conditions, the treatment in question has been shown to be more effective than patients treated in some other way, typically referred to as a "treatment-as-usual" (or placebo) condition.

I do not want to undermine the value of evidence-based treatments in general, but a quick comment to parents here about "under controlled conditions." Efficacy studies (research that is conducted to determine if a treatment is effective and, if so, to what extent), have had their share of criticism. For example, John List, a distinguished service professor in economics at the University of Chicago, is a strong voice in a movement known as *implementation science,* or the science of "scaling up." List describes what he refers to as a "voltage drop," ideas that can look good in a small, tightly controlled environment, but when the idea is implemented on a larger scale, the treatment results often do not hold up (List, 2022).

For example, cognitive behavioral therapy (CBT), developed by the late psychiatrist Aaron Beck, has substantial research support (see Chapter 6 for a full description of CBT and its supporting evidence). I have no doubt that had I been able to see Dr. Beck in therapy, I would have received excellent CBT. I would feel equally confident that I could also receive high-quality CBT from one of the other many well-trained, certified, and experienced CBT therapists throughout the world. However, a less experienced therapist, maybe one who received a smattering of CBT in graduate school (me, for example), or maybe one who attended a weekend course in CBT? Not so much. So, yes, the movement toward trying to scientifically establish what treatments are effective is a great thing, but I think it is important for parents to know that even the best-studied and validated treatments might be disappointing when delivered in a watered-down manner that substantially reduces their voltage.

To illustrate the point, I am going to pick on dialectical behavior therapy (DBT). DBT has become almost ubiquitous in psychotherapy, but despite substantial empirical support for the treatment of patients who are prone to emotional dysregulation and self-harming behaviors, it is likely highly susceptible to a voltage drop. DBT, as it was originally developed

by Marsha Linehan at the University of Washington, consists of four essential treatment components: Weekly or ideally twice-weekly individual
therapy; a weekly two-hour skills training group; a therapist consultation
group; and after-hours availability of the therapist to the patient (Linehan,
1993). As it turns out, the last three components of DBT are difficult to
pull off for most therapists, especially those in private practice. Most
therapists cannot organize and implement skills training in a group
format, so in most cases, skills are woven into the individual sessions. This
is not ideal because, even in a weekly group format devoted just to
teaching DBT skills, it takes a full year to teach all of them. Participating
in a therapist consultation group (reviewing cases with other therapists) is
challenging as well because one must find other willing therapists in order
to participate in such a group—not an easy task. Finally, regarding after-
hours availability, not all therapists are willing to offer this to patients as it
can be quite stressful and draining.

I have long suspected that many therapists who say they provide DBT in
actuality probably do not, given how difficult it is to implement all four
essential components. To satisfy my own curiosity, I gathered some data
on this to see what I could learn. I put together a short SurveyMonkey that
I posted on various Facebook groups for therapists asking if they would
be willing to complete it. The first screening question on the survey was,
"Are you a therapist who currently uses DBT as a routine part of your
psychotherapy practice?" If the answer was "yes," the person could then
move on to complete the survey. The remaining questions were straightforward, such as: "Do you participate in a DBT consultation group?",
"Are you routinely available to your DBT clients for a phone or text
consultation after hours?", and so on.

I received a total of 48 completed surveys, and, among those, only
10.4% of respondents (five therapists) were providing all four essential
components of DBT. Well, what if a little bit of DBT is better than none at
all? The problem with this is we simply do not know, because all of the
research supporting the efficacy of DBT is based on delivering all four
components, and therefore we can draw no conclusions about the value in
offering patients something other than that. I am sure someone would be
able to design a more scientifically rigorous study than I did, and I would
encourage them to do so. However, as a preliminary finding, I think it is
pretty telling that almost 90% of therapists in my sample who say they are
providing DBT really are not. Similarly, I might also question the value of
a treatment that is so difficult to implement in real-world practice.

Similarly, along the lines of transparency, I think psychiatrists and
pharmaceutical companies need quite a bit of work in this area as well. I
cannot tell you how many times a parent has said to me, "If we could only
find the right medication for my child." While medication is often helpful

for people with more serious forms of mental illness (again, bipolar disorder and schizophrenia), I think most parents would be shocked at the research on the efficacy of psychotropic medications, which calls into question whether they really do anything at all.

For example, consider what we know about the efficacy of antidepressants. In a recent study, Marc Stone and his colleagues examined data submitted by drug companies to the U.S. Food and Drug Administration between 1979–2016. The data set was massive: 73,338 depressed patients who participated in a total of 232 randomized, placebo-controlled trials that were either prescribed an antidepressant or a placebo (Stone et al., 2022). (A placebo is an inert substance that has no active chemical properties.) Results from their analyses indicated that for 85% of the patients, antidepressants performed no better than placebo. Well, what about the remaining 15%; it helped them right? Not really. On a scale that measures the severity of depressive symptoms that has a maximum score of 52 points, those patients' scores improved by an average of only 1.75 points, a difference so slight as to be clinically meaningless. Scores for children improved by less than one point (0.71). If you are a parent, please do not interpret this to mean you should take your child off their antidepressant medication. Some people do get better on antidepressants. However, the data suggests that this improvement may be more likely due to the placebo effect rather than the chemical properties of the medication. The takeaway here is just that the medical community and the pharmaceutical companies would have us believe antidepressants are far more helpful than they actually are.

For an excellent (and terrifying) discussion of the history of psychotropic medication, the role that pharmaceutical companies have played in public perception of the effectiveness of medication, as well as the research on medication efficacy itself, I would refer the reader to *Desperate Remedies: Psychiatry's Turbulent Quest to Cure Mental Illness* (Scull, 2022).

For school counselors, capitalize on parents far more often, and, despite good intentions, be wary of interventions used on campus that are counterproductive to building resilience. Schools in the U.S. are now tasked with the responsibility of addressing the epidemic of children and teens presenting on campus with mental health challenges. How and to what degree this challenge is being met likely varies by region, but, in my part of the country, every school I know is struggling with how to best help students with depression, anxiety, and self-harming behaviors. School shootings have also increased pressure on school administrators and staff to pay much more careful attention to students who might be at risk for violence.

In my experience of interacting with school counselors, I believe they often suffer the same fate as individual therapists in the community in that far too much attention is being paid to what's happening on the inside of kids and not enough on the outside. Individual counseling sessions are provided again as if there is something wrong inside the student that needs correcting. In the same way that individual therapists lack the power to successfully disrupt and mitigate external, situational variables that are affecting the child's well-being, this is the case as well for school counselors and therapists. It also does not seem like much work is being done with parents, but incorporating some family work into these sessions would likely benefit the student and allow the school therapist to impact areas of the student's life that could not be done otherwise.

Furthermore, rather than addressing mental health challenges by working with children and teens one at a time, schools are missing out on a golden opportunity to positively impact a much larger number of students in a far more efficient manner.

Schools have direct access to parents, and, as I have discussed throughout this book, parents are the best possible agents of change in that they can implement helpful interventions at home. I recommend that schools consider conducting a series of workshops and inviting parents to attend. Most parents are worried about their child's mental health, and they are hungry for information so that they can better address their child's emotional struggles. The topics of the workshops would include the interventions and strategies outlined in this chapter for parents. For example, many parents are only vaguely familiar with the research on screen time and how it affects depression and anxiety, and I would imagine that they would greatly appreciate learning how to reduce their child's screen time or how to better monitor their online activity without a fight.

Many school counselors are good at what they do and very well-intentioned, but some of the interventions I have seen implemented on school campuses have a good probability of making kids more dependent and even less resilient. For example, many of the teenagers I have worked with have a plan already in place as to what to do if they struggle during the school day. Typically, the plan entails going to the counseling office for support. Often, the student knows they have permission just to leave class when they feel it necessary, and teachers are also encouraged to send students to the counseling office as well. In many cases, when a student is having difficulty, the school will call the parents and ask that they be picked up. At first glance, this makes sense: Provide the necessary mental health support when the students need it.

However, knowing what we do about escape/avoidant behaviors, we can see why a student having the ability to leave the classroom might inadvertently reinforce these behaviors. If something reduces my stress and makes me feel better, I am very likely going to make use of that thing again. For example, when one of my patients was becoming anxious in class, he was told he could leave the classroom with his best friend, and they could hang out together outside until he was feeling better. The problems with this "intervention" are obvious. (Interestingly, and quite rightly so, after our conversations in session about how we can inadvertently reinforce the wrong thing, the boy's mother learned about this in a parent-teacher meeting, saw the problem with it right away, and put a stop to it.) Furthermore, if going to the counseling center is at the top of a student's mental health plan, it sends the subtle message that they lack the capacity to remain in and successfully cope with moderately stressful, albeit age-appropriate situations.

I think it would be far more helpful for the student's mental health plan to foster resiliency and independence. It is fine for them to leave class to go see a therapist, but I recommend making the time spent in the counseling office as brief as possible. The focus should be on encouraging what might be hard for the student, i.e., going back to class and tolerating their distress, and reminding them that the therapist is confident of their ability to do so. The only way something stops being hard for us is when we practice it over and over until it isn't hard anymore.

Recommendations for Insurance Companies

Become knowledgeable about, and capitalize on, the almost 40 years of research documenting the efficacy of family therapy. Problems this addresses: Prolonging a child and family's suffering needlessly and making their mental health condition worse. In my experience, insurance companies are woefully behind the times when it comes to being familiar with, and paying for, family-based treatments. I cannot remember a single instance of communicating with an insurance company in which the subject of family therapy came up without my raising it. I also do not ever recall any of the families that I have worked with who have been advised by their insurance company to seek out family therapy.

Insurance companies are subject to the same inherent bias from which the rest of the mental health community suffers: Pushing for individual therapy and other treatments directed solely at the child. I am certain that insurance companies are reeling from the now-decade-long surge in children and adolescents needing mental health care, and they are surely looking for ways to meet this demand while at the same time managing their costs. It would seem highly advantageous, therefore, to more fully understand the research on the efficacy of family therapy and promote its use as a matter of course. Regarding cost savings, as mentioned in Chapter 4, I would direct an insurance company's attention to the work of D. Russell Crane and Jacob Christenson (2012), which summarizes the results of 22 studies indicating that family therapy, relative to just individual therapy, results in a significant reduction of healthcare costs.

Assign a care advocate to families to keep patients from being shuffled from one unhelpful treatment to another. Problems this addresses: Same as above.

The mental health community is quite compartmentalized, as is the health insurance industry, to the detriment of children and families. Children with serious conditions who are not getting better tend to be bumped from one ineffective treatment to another without any consideration of the big picture, thus making their condition worse. More problematic still, desperate parents are given recommendations for treatment that will probably not do their child much good at all (for example, yet another individual therapist or one more IOP program).

It would be highly useful for insurance companies to routinely assign some sort of patient or services advocate to families with high-risk children. Some do, but in my experience, most do not. To complicate the matter further, when an insurance company does provide an advocate, that person's recommendations are influenced by obvious conflicts of interests, i.e., to find treatment options, yes, but at the lowest cost possible. Advocates could be far more effective if they are given the freedom and latitude to make truly independent decisions and not feel their job is in jeopardy if they do.

Consider incentivizing family therapists so that there are more of us. Problem this addresses: Family therapist scarcity.

For reasons that I have never understood, some insurance companies reimburse less for an hour of family therapy than an hour of individual therapy. Family therapy is much harder and a lot more stressful, but in many cases far more useful. It requires a unique skill set that not every therapist possesses. And, because it is more difficult, not many therapists want to do it. For these reasons, there simply are not enough of us to go around, but incentives could help change that. Family therapy should not be paid at a lower rate relative to individual therapy, or better still, family therapists should be paid at a rate that is commensurate with their skill level and the potential cost savings they bring to the insurance company.

Parents are scared, so treat them like human beings. I cannot begin to describe the amount of suffering I have witnessed inflicted on families by the actions of insurance companies here in the U.S.

Not all insurance companies, of course. In many instances, I have had the pleasure of working with insurance companies that are professional, compassionate, and committed to helping families obtain much-needed treatment.

The others, however, are horrendous. It is clear to me that their number one priority, well above doing the right thing, is to enhance their own financial bottom line. There is a "healthcare" company in the area in which I practice that has been slapped many times by the courts for providing inadequate mental health treatment to its members. I have been a witness to its putting family after family through the meat grinder, denying much-needed treatment or offering useless treatments to parents who want nothing more than to help their child get proper care. The pain that these families experience is indescribable. If you are a parent reading this, you likely can attest to what I am saying about insurance companies, and I am guessing you too have endured delays in care, stonewalling, condescension, and callous indifference. This needs to stop.

Some Final Thoughts

The reader will probably note that none of the strategies or interventions discussed in this chapter includes hiring more therapists. This is the remedy that I hear most often proposed, and I do see a certain logic in it. A great number of young people are struggling, so who better to help them than therapists? Yes, of course, we need enough therapists so that anyone who needs help can get it.

However, this solution is incomplete as it does nothing to reverse the increased trend of mental health problems and the corresponding demand for ever more therapists. To respond to the mental health crisis only by hiring more therapists is what Joel Brockner (1992) refers to as an "escalation of commitment to a failing course of action," the tendency to double down on a solution that clearly is not working. In the case of adolescent mental illness, responding to the crisis by mobilizing more therapists is an attempt to address the demand, but it does nothing to address the underlying problems that are creating the demand in the first place.

One can liken this approach to trying to reduce the problem of gun violence in the U.S. by hiring more emergency room physicians. It makes much more sense to me to focus on solutions that identify the underlying causes of increased mental illness in young people, and then implement community-based strategies that stand a decent chance of keeping kids out of the therapist's office altogether.

The strategies and interventions outlined throughout this book, and in this chapter in particular, are all entirely doable. Each stands a chance of at least partially improving the current situation. However, taken collectively, I believe the changes that I am proposing in the treatment of child and adolescent mental health challenges stand an excellent chance of making a difference. I am reasonably confident of this because, when my colleagues and I implement these strategies, we see the positive results of this every day.

It is an honor and privilege for me to sit with families in what is almost certain to be one of the darkest periods of their lives. The child they knew who was once loving and innocent often in no way resembles the angry, depressed, and uncommunicative person living under their roof right now.

Despite all of their best efforts to help, parents have no idea how their family has gotten so far off track and they have even less of an idea as to what to do about it. They are to blame, or so they think, because that is the message our culture sends: *When kids are messed up, it's the parents' fault.*

Sometimes, of course, yes, but most of the time fault lies in families where the parents are abusive and the mistreatment of their child is obvious. However, most parents are not abusive, yet their child or teen is still clearly struggling. Almost every parent I know, myself included, wouldn't hesitate to throw themselves in front of a train if they knew it would save their child's life. Blaming parents is also still alive and well in the mental health community. Recently, a new treatment program opened in my area, and, while at a cocktail party, I happened to be talking to one of the principal developers of the program. I asked them how parents would be included in their teen's treatment, and what model of family therapy they would be implementing. Their response? *"Well, you know what these parents are like."* (Actually, as a matter of fact, I do. They're amazing.) It is time we let go of blaming parents, which does nothing but add more shame and misery to their lives.

And, on the kids' side of things, they certainly have no idea how they got to be this way either. When you ask them why they are depressed, anxious, or thinking about suicide, they will often give you an answer, but as anyone who has worked with these kids knows, the answers are very dissatisfying and often don't add up very well. That's because they really don't know—their words are just an attempt to explain something that is often well outside of their awareness or understanding. How can a kid put words to situational influences, emotional or behavioral contagion, classification, and crowding-out effects, the unintended consequences of helicopter parenting, or low mood precipitated by excessive screen time? In the same way that their parents can't explain it, neither can the kid, but they are being honest when they say they're unhappy. They are relying on us, the adults, to figure out what is happening to them, and have the wisdom, compassion, and expertise to alleviate their suffering.

Given the severity of the current mental health crisis and the fact that it shows no signs of remitting, it is time that all of us collectively—parents, providers, and the community—rethink what we are doing.

We can do better, and we must.

References

Brockner, J. (1992). The escalation of commitment to a failing course of action: Toward theoretical progress. *The Academy of Management Review, 17*(1), 39–61. 10.2307/258647

Crane, D. R., & Christenson, J. D. (2012). A summary report of the cost-effectiveness of the profession and practice of marriage and family therapy. *Contemporary Family Therapy: An International Journal, 34*(2), 204–216. 10.1007/s10591-012-9187-5

Linehan, M. M. (1993). *Cognitive-behavioral treatment of borderline personality disorder* (1st ed.). The Guilford Press.

List, J. A. (2022). *The voltage effect: How to make good ideas great and great ideas scale.* Currency.

Meehl, P. E. (1973). Why I do not attend case conferences. In *Psychodiagnosis: Selected papers* (pp. 225–304). University of Minnesota Press.

O'Sullivan, S. (2021). *The sleeping beauties: And other stories of mystery illness.* Pantheon.

Scull, A. (2022). *Desperate remedies: Psychiatry's turbulent quest to cure mental illness.* The Belknap Press of Harvard University Press.

Stone, M. B., Yaseen, Z. S., Miller, B. J., Richardville, K., Kalaria, S. N., & Kirsch, I. (2022). Response to acute monotherapy for major depressive disorder in randomized, placebo controlled trials submitted to the U.S. Food and Drug Administration: Individual participant data analysis. *The BMJ, 378*, Article e067606. 10.1136/bmj-2021-067606

Index

Page numbers in *italics* indicate figures; page numbers in **bold** indicate tables.

bubonic plague 23
bullying 13
Burns, David 99

CAFFI *See* Child & Adolescent Family
    Functioning Inventory (CAFFI)
case examples: anxious avoidance 167,
    200–216; self-harm 97,
    146–163
Casline, Elizabeth 179
CBT *See* cognitive behavior
    therapy (CBT)
celebrity suicides 27–28
cell phones: anxious avoidance and
    181–183; effects of 10–13,
    32–35; mitigating the negative
    effects of 220–223; monitoring
    for safety 109–110, 223; use
    during COVID-19 pandemic 15
Child & Adolescent Family
    Functioning Inventory (CAFFI)
    161–162, *162*, *163*, 214,
    215, *216*
child and adolescent, mental health:
    anxiety in 168–169; cognitive
    behavior therapy 99–102;
    dialectical behavior therapy
    102–104; digital technology,
    effects of 10–13; 18-item,
    research-informed strategy for
    219–237, **221**; family therapy
    (*See* family-based treatments);
    overview 1–6; prevalence of 9;
    rise in, causes and contributing
    factors 9–16; self-injury 26–27,
    35; smartphones, effect of
    10–13, 32–35; social contagion
    21–28, 34; suicide attempts
    (*See* suicide ideation and
    attempts); temperament, role of
    78–80. *See also* Intensive
    Family-Focused Therapy (IFFT)
Christakis, Nicholas 23
Christenson, Jacob 60, 234
Cialdini, Robert 43
classification effect 53, 224, 228
Cline, Foster 29
clinical language 52
cognitive behavior therapy (CBT):
    history 99; outcome studies on
    101–102; self-harm and 102;

strategies 101; treatment
    components 99–100
cognitive distortions 99–100
communication patterns 47
coping strategies 43
cost-effective, family therapy
    60–61, 234
COVID-19 pandemic: anxious
    avoidance and 168, 169;
    functional tic-like disorder
    (FTLD) 24–25; impact on
    mental health 14–15; induced
    social isolation 9, 14, 15, 167;
    phones and social media
    use 15
Crane, D. Russell 60, 234
creativity and persistence 171
*The Crowd: A Study of the Popular
    Mind* 22
crowding out effect 33, 87, 181,
    222, 237
Curtis, Nicola 69
cyberbullying 13
cybervictimization 13

Darley, John 84
DBT *See* dialectical behavior
    therapy (DBT)
"depressed" (use of the word) 55
depression: *versus* anger 107–109;
    social contagion and 25–26;
    social media use 12
*Desperate Remedies: Psychiatry's
    Turbulent Quest to Cure
    Mental Illness* 232
deviance training 84
device-free time periods 222–223
*Diagnostic and Statistical Manual of
    Mental Disorders* (DSM) 228
dialectical behavior therapy (DBT) 90,
    91, 102–103, 230–231; history
    102; outcomes studies 104;
    parasuicidal behavior 103–104;
    self-harm and 104; treatment
    components 102–103
Diamond, Gary 70, 138
Diamond, Guy 70, 138
"difficult" temperaments 78
difficult-to-parent child 66, 79, 86,
    148, 225
digital drugs 10–11. *See also* smartphones

therapy 122–134; as it relates to
the family 135–137; cellphone
and 47–48; not related to family
137–138; parent therapy
138–141; parents responding to
112–114; social contagion and
26–27, 35. See also nonsuicidal
self-injury; suicide ideation and
attempts
session content and clinical objectives:
expected course of treatment
141–142; family-based
treatments 134–138; helpful
treatment components
142–143; individual therapy
122–134; parent therapy
138–141; skills training 141
Sexton, Thomas 66
Shahtahmasebi, Said 9
"should" statements 100
siblings, bidirectional resonance
82–83, 83
situational influences 84–85, 220,
226, 237
skills training: anxious avoidance
193–194; self-harm 141
sleep duration: electronic device use
and 11–12, 33; social network
and 22–23
The Sleeping Beauties: And Other
Stories of Mystery Illness
25, 229
smartphones: anxious avoidance and
181–183; effect of 10–13,
32–35; mitigating the negative
effects of 220–223; monitoring
for safety 109–110, 223; use
during COVID-19 pandemic 15
social comparison 11
social contagion: anxiety and 26;
defined 22; depression and
25–26; hikikomori and 168;
hypothesis 21–22, 34; mass
psychogenic illness 23–25;
media on suicide attempts
27–28; self-injury and 26–27;
social networks and 22–23
social disintegration hypothesis 21
social isolation, COVID-induced 9, 14,
15, 43, 167

social media 11, 12; bullying and 13;
use during COVID-19
pandemic 15
social networks and contagion
22–23, 222
social proof 43
space-time clusters 28
Srivastav, Deepika 29
Steinberg, L. 26
suicidal and self-harming kids, IFFT
and 77
suicide clusters 28–29
suicide ideation and attempts: bullying
and 13; celebrity suicides
27–28; cognitive behavior
therapy 99–102; COVID-19
pandemic and 14–15; dialectical
behavior therapy 102–104;
family functioning and 63, 64,
65; hanging, death by 20; in
male population 20–21; media
on suicide attempts 27–28;
Micronesia 20–21; online
suicide-related searches 15;
parasuicidal behavior 103–104;
prevalence of 98; social
contagion hypothesis (See social
contagion). See also nonsuicidal
self-injury
suicide rates: LGBTQ+ youth 10;
younger girls 10
systematic desensitization 172
Szapocznik, José 69

"talk-it-to-death" strategy 51
tantrum 46
team-based approach, IFFT 88–90
technology-based behaviors 11
temperament: anxious avoidance and
174; role 78–80
tetanus vaccination 24
"The Hidden Influence of Social
Networks" 23
tic-like symptoms 24–25
TikTok videos 43
The Tipping Point 20
Tourette syndrome 24
transdiagnostic (IFFT) 76, 77
"trauma" (use of the word) 54–55,
224, 225
Trevor Project 10

tug-of-war 50, 81
Twenge, Jean 29, 32

vocabulary 51
voltage drop 229, 230

Warren County High School
    (McMinnville, Tennessee) 24

well-being 21
word choice 52, *55*
"wounded pride" 20

Youth Outcomes Questionnaire
    (Y-OQ2.01) 160–161, *161*,
    214, *215*

For Product Safety Concerns and Information please contact our EU
representative GPSR@taylorandfrancis.com
Taylor & Francis Verlag GmbH, Kaufingerstraße 24, 80331 München, Germany